ORTHOPAEDIC
POCKET
PROCEDURES

SPORTS MEDICINE

NOTICE

ORTHOPAEDIC POCKET PROCEDURES

SPORTS MEDICINE

ROBERT A. ARCIERO, MD

University of Connecticut School of Medicine
Farmington, Connecticut

Series Editor

COURTLAND G. LEWIS, MD

University of Connecticut School of Medicine
Farmington, Connecticut

Illustrator

TIMOTHY E. HENGST

McGRAW-HILL
MEDICAL PUBLISHING DIVISION
New York   Chicago   San Francisco
Lisbon   London   Madrid   Mexico City   Milan
New Delhi   San Juan   Seoul   Singapore
Sydney   Toronto

Orthopaedic Pocket Procedures: GENERAL ORTHOPAEDICS
Copyright © 2004 by The **McGraw-Hill Companies**, Inc. All rights reserved. Printed in the United States of America. Except as permitted under the United States Copyright Act of 1976, no part of this publication may be reproduced or distributed in any form or by any means, or stored in a data base or retrieval system, without the prior written permission of the publisher.

1 2 3 4 5 6 7 8 9 0 DOC/DOC 0 9 8 7 6 5 4 3

ISBN   0-07-136989-9

This book was set in Times Roman by PV&M Publishing Solutions.
The editors were Darlene Cooke, Lisa Silverman, and Karen Davis.
The production supervisor was Catherine Saggese.
The interior text designer was Marsha Cohen/Parallelogram.
The cover designer was John Vairo.
The index was prepared by Robert Swanson.
RR Donnelley was printer and binder.

This book is printed on acid-free paper.

Library of Congress Cataloging-in-Publication Data

Arciero, Robert A.
    Sports medicine / Robert Arciero; illustrator, Timothy E. Hengst.
        p. cm.   (Orthopaedic pocket procedures)
    Includes bibliographical references and index.
    ISBN 0-07-136989-9 (softcover)
        1. Sports injuries—Patients—Rehabilitation—Handbooks, manuals, etc. 2. Wounds and injuries—Surgery—Handbooks, manuals, etc. 3. Sports medicine—Handbooks, manuals, etc.   I. Title. II. Series.
    [DNLM: 1. Athletic Injuries—surgery—Handbooks. 2. Athletic Injuries—rehabilitation—Handbooks. 3. Orthopedic Procedures—Handbooks. 4. Physical Therapy Techniques—Handbooks. QT 29 A674s 2003]

    RD97.A24 2003
    617.1'027--dc21   2003044472

CONTENTS

PART III KNEE

CONTENTS

IN ALPHABETICAL ORDER

PREFACE

The Sports Medicine edition of *Orthopaedic Pocket Procedures* provides a succinct, user-friendly resource that is practical and informative. This book is a handy reference of sports medicine procedures featuring CPT codes coupled with the ICD-9 codes, surgical indications, alternative treatments, and synopses of surgical approaches and pertinent anatomy. Most procedures are represented with diagrams and illustrations to provide additional understanding. Further, procedure chapters include several timely references and note-taking space to jot down surgeon preferences and details unique to the particular case. All of this is presented in a snapshot, spread-page format for expedient usage.

This publication represents the surgical case-log and collective experience of sports-medicine experts and has been compiled to illustrate commonly performed sports medicine procedures as well as innovative and newer arthroscopic techniques. Orthopaedic residents, operating room personnel, and young orthopaedists in their early career will find this an easily accessible resource.

Whether you are an orthopaedic resident, an orthopaedist recently in practice, a physical therapist, an athletic trainer, or other health-care professional, we hope that this resource will serve as a timely reference providing expedient information and a stimulus for more in-depth learning. This work was developed by sports-medicine clinicians for clinicians, and we hope that it will provide useful advice and insight to those who care for active patients.

ROBERT A. ARCIERO, MD
Farmington, Connecticut
September 2003

CONTRIBUTORS

SHOULDER

KEVIN P. SHEA, MD

Associate Professor of Orthopaedics
University of Connecticut Health Center
Farmington, Connecticut

KNEE

CARL W. NISSEN, MD

Assistant Professor of Orthopaedics
University of Connecticut Health Center
Farmington, Connecticut

FOOT/ANKLE

DEAN C. TAYLOR, MD, LTC, MC

Department of Orthopaedics
Keller Army Hospital
West Point, New York

To Cathy,
wife, mother, companion for life.
You are the pillar of our family and your selfless sacrifice has
allowed all of us to thrive and has been an
inspiration to all who know you. . . .

PART I

SHOULDER

REMOVAL OF CALCIFIC DEPOSITS

CPT code   23000 removal of subdeltoid or intratendinous calcific deposits

ICD-9 code   726.11 calcifying tendonitis of the shoulder

INDICATIONS

Pain and restricted movement of the shoulder due to calcifying tendonitis of the rotator cuff tendons, not responsive to nonsteroidal anti-inflammatory drugs (NSAIDs), rehabilitation, or subacromial steroid injections.

ALTERNATIVE TREATMENTS

* arthroscopic debridement of calcific tendonitis
* barbotage (recurrent piercing with a needle)
* direct steroid injection into calcified tendon

SURGICAL ANATOMY

Incision
* deltoid splitting

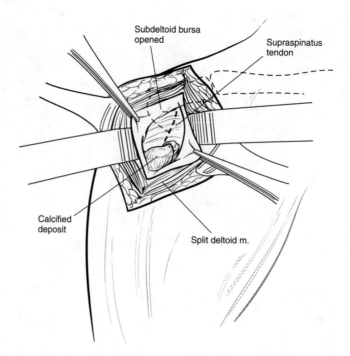

APPROACHES

Surgical Techniques

- deltoid-splitting incision
- avoid axillary nerve (4 cm distal to acromial margin)
- identify calcific nodule(s)
- incise tendon in line with fibers
- scrape out calcium
- repair tendon side-to-side
- layered closure

POSTOPERATIVE MANAGEMENT

- sling for comfort
- cryotherapy
- pendulum exercises day 1

REHABILITATION

- passive range of motion (ROM) until comfortable
- active-assisted and active ROM
- rotator cuff and scapular strengthening

COMPLICATIONS

- recurrent pain
- inadequate removal of calcium
- loss of motion

SELECTED REFERENCES

Utoff HK, Sarkar K. Calcifying tendonitis in the shoulder. In: Matsen FA , Rockwood CA, eds. The shoulder. Philadelphia: WB Saunders, 1990:774–788.

Jerosch J, Strauss JM, Schmiel S. Arthroscopic treatment of calcific tendonitis of the shoulder. J Shoulder Elbow Surg 1998;7(1):30–37.

NOTES

_____
_____
_____
_____
_____
_____

PARTIAL CLAVICULECTOMY, DISTAL

CPT code   23120 partial claviculectomy (distal)

ICD-9 codes   715.11 osteoarthrosis, localized to the shoulder (unspecified site)
                      716.11 traumatic arthropathy of the shoulder (unspecified site)
                      831.04 acromioclavicular joint dislocation
                      840.0 acromioclavicular joint sprain

INDICATIONS

Pain and limitation of motion secondary to derangement of the acromio-clavicular (AC) joint, nonresponsive to NSAIDs or intra-articular injection of steroids.

ALTERNATIVE TREATMENTS

- intra-articular injection of steroids
- arthroscopic resection of distal clavicle

SURGICAL ANATOMY

Incision
- transverse or Saber

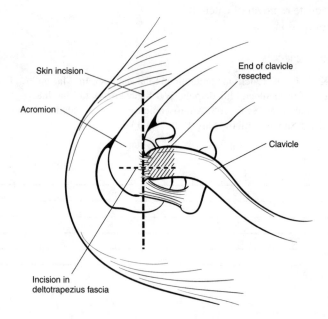

APPROACHES

Surgical Techniques

- skin incision
- split fascia longitudinally over lateral clavicle
- expose distal clavicle
- resect 1–2 cm distal to clavicle using power saw
- file superior cortex
- close fascia
- layered skin closure

POSTOPERATIVE MANAGEMENT

- sling for comfort
- cryotherapy

REHABILITATION

- pendulum exercises
- active-assisted and active ROM
- shoulder strengthening
- return to sport when full range of motion (FROM) and strength achieved (4–6 weeks)

COMPLICATIONS

- failure to relieve pain
- instability of distal clavicle
- inadequate resection

SELECTED REFERENCES

Mumford EB. Acromioclavicular dislocation. J Bone Joint Surg Am 1941;23:799–802.
Shaffer BS. Painful conditions of the acromioclavicular joint. J Am Acad Orthop Surg 1999;7(3):176–188.

NOTES

_____

_____

_____

_____

_____

_____

_____

PARTIAL CLAVICULECTOMY, PROXIMAL

CPT code	23120 partial claviculectomy (proximal)
ICD-9 codes	715.11 osteoarthrosis, localized to the shoulder (unspecified site)
	716.11 traumatic arthropathy of the shoulder (unspecified site)
	718.31 chronic dislocation, shoulder

INDICATIONS

Pain, swelling, and limitation of motion secondary to derangement of the sternoclavicular joint, nonresponsive to NSAIDs or activity modification.

ALTERNATIVE TREATMENT

• continued conservative management

SURGICAL ANATOMY

Incision
• transverse incision inferior to sternoclavicular joint

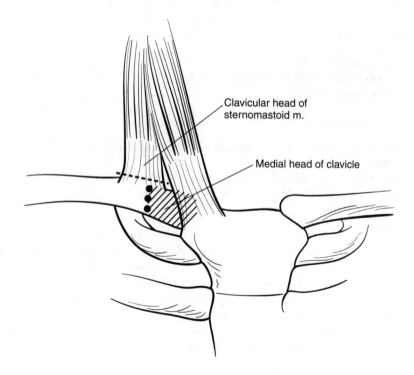

Clavicular head of sternomastoid m.

Medial head of clavicle

APPROACH

Surgical Techniques
- skin incision
- split fascia longitudinally over medial clavicle
- detach clavicular head of sternomastoid muscle
- evaluate stability—may need to reconstruct costoclavicular ligaments with subclavius or fascia lata
- insert retractor behind medial clavicle
- multiple drill holes medial to costoclavicular ligaments
- osteotomize clavicle—remove medial end
- file bone smooth
- reattach sternomastoid muscle
- layered skin closure

POSTOPERATIVE MANAGEMENT

- sling for comfort
- cryotherapy

REHABILITATION

- pendulum exercises
- active-assisted and active ROM
- shoulder strengthening
- return to sport when FROM and strength achieved (4–6 weeks)

COMPLICATIONS

- injury to great vessels
- instability, recurrent pain

SELECTED REFERENCES

Rockwood CA. Disorders of the sternoclavicular joint. In: Rockwood RA, Matsen FA, eds. The shoulder. Philadelphia: WB Saunders, 1990:477–525.
Pingsmann A, Patsalis T, Michiels I. Resection arthroplasty of the sternoclavicular joint for primary degenerative sternoclavicular arthritis. J Bone Joint Surg Br 2002;84:513–517.

NOTES

_____
_____
_____
_____
_____

ACROMIOPLASTY WITH CORACOACROMIAL LIGAMENT RELEASE

CPT code   23130 acromioplasty with coracoacromial ligament release

ICD-9 codes   726.10 disorders of bursae and tendons in the shoulder region—unspecified
                  727.61 rotator cuff rupture (complete tear)
                  840.4   rotator cuff strain (partial tear)

INDICATIONS

Pain and limitation of motion secondary to impingement of the rotator cuff tendon(s) by the coracoacromial arch that does not respond to at least 3 months of rehabilitation, NSAIDs, and subacromial steroid injections.

ALTERNATIVE TREATMENTS

- arthroscopic acromioplasty
- rotator cuff repair
- arthroscopic bursectomy

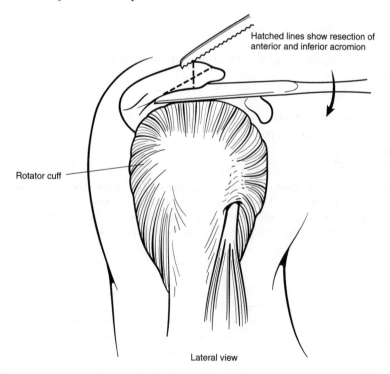

Hatched lines show resection of anterior and inferior acromion

Rotator cuff

Lateral view

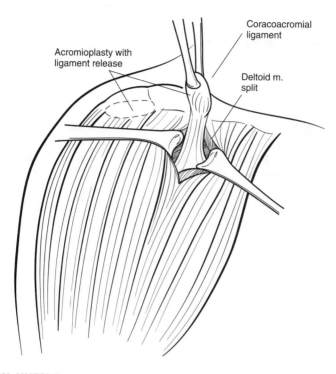

Coracoacromial ligament

Acromioplasty with ligament release

Deltoid m. split

SURGICAL ANATOMY

Incision
- Saber incision in Langer's lines

APPROACHES

Surgical Techniques
- supine or modified beach chair position
- surgical incision
- split or detach deltoid muscle
- identify coracoacromial ligament
- ¾ inch osteotome to remove acromial spur
- rasp bone smooth
- reattach deltoid with sutures through bone
- skin closure

POSTOPERATIVE MANAGEMENT

- sling for comfort

REHABILITATION

- active-assisted and passive motion
- rotator cuff strengthening
- return to sport in 6–12 weeks

SELECTED REFERENCES

Neer CS II. Anterior acromioplasty for the chronic impingement syndrome in the shoulder. J Bone Joint Surg Am 1972;54:41–50.

Tibone JE, Jobe FW, Kerlan RK, Carter VS. Shoulder impingement syndrome in athletes treated by anterior acromioplasty. Clin Orthop 1985;198:134–137.

NOTES

OSTECTOMY OF SCAPULA, PARTIAL

CPT code   23190 ostectomy of the scapula, partial, for snapping scapula syndrome

ICD-9 codes   726.10 disorders of bursae and tendons in the shoulder region—unspecified
                    726.2   other affections of the shoulder region, not elsewhere classified

INDICATIONS

Painful crepitus or snapping emanating from the superior medial angle of the scapula, nonresponsive to at least 3 months of rehabilitation, NSAIDs, and steroid injections.

ALTERNATIVE TREATMENT

- arthroscopic subscapular bursectomy

SURGICAL ANATOMY

Incision
- parallel to medial scapular spine

APPROACHES

Surgical Techniques
- prone position
- incision as shown in parallel to medial border of scapula
- elevate trapezius from scapular spine
- subperiosteal elevation of supraspinatus, rhomboids, and levator scapulae from scapula
- resect superior medial angle with motorized saw
- reapproximate supraspinatus to scapular spine through drill holes
- skin closure

POSTOPERATIVE MANAGEMENT

- sling for comfort

REHABILITATION

- passive motion, immediately
- active motion at 8 weeks
- strengthening exercises at 12 weeks
- return to sport in 4–6 months

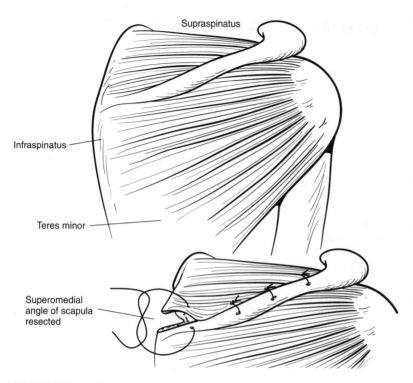

Supraspinatus

Infraspinatus

Teres minor

Superomedial
angle of scapula
resected

SELECTED REFERENCES

Kuhn JE, Plancher KD, Hawkins RJ. Symptomatic scapulothoracic crepitus and bursitis. J Am Acad Orthop Surg 1998;6:267–273.

Sisto DJ, Jobe FW. The operative treatment of scapulothoracic bursitis in professional pitchers. Am J Sports Med 1986;14:192–194.

NOTES

_____

_____

_____

_____

_____

_____

_____

_____

_____

_____

_____

_____

TENOTOMY, LONG TENDON OF BICEPS

CPT code   **23405 tenotomy of the long tendon of biceps**

ICD-9 code(s)   **726.12 biceps tenosynovitis**

INDICATIONS

Pain, weakness, and limitation of motion due to chronic biceps tendonitis or recurrent subluxation of the biceps tendon that does not respond to rehabilitation, NSAIDs, or steroid injections.

ALTERNATIVE TREATMENTS

- arthroscopic tenotomy
- biceps tenodesis

Incision

- deltopectoral or arthroscopic

APPROACHES

Surgical Techniques

- deltopectoral approach
- identify bicipital groove
- open tendon sheath, place traction suture into biceps tendon
- deliver as much tendon from intra-articular space as possible and transect the tendon (note: tenotomy can be performed arthroscopically)

POSTOPERATIVE MANAGEMENT

- sling for comfort

REHABILITATION

- active-assisted and passive ROM, immediately
- strengthening for 4–6 weeks
- return to sport in 6–12 weeks

COMPLICATIONS

- continued pain
- cosmetic deformity with distal biceps muscle

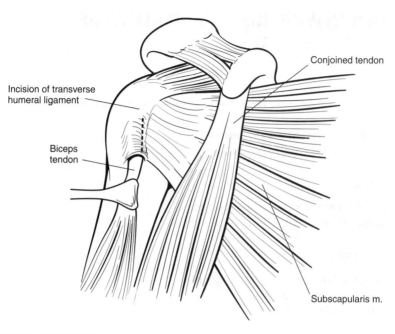

SELECTED REFERENCES

Sethi N, Wright R, Yamaguchi K. Disorders of the long head of the biceps tendon.
   J Shoulder Elbow Surg 1999;8:644–654.
Gill TJ, McIrvin E, Mair SD, Hawkins, RJ. Results of biceps tenotomy for the treatment of pathology of the long head of the biceps brachii. J Shoulder Elbow Surg
   2001;10:247–249.

NOTES

OPEN REPAIR, RUPTURED ROTATOR CUFF TENDONS

CPT codes   23410, 23412, 23420 open repair of ruptured rotator cuff tendons
23410 acute, 23412 chronic, 23420 complete including acromioplasty

ICD-9 code   727.61 torn rotator cuff (complete)
840.4 torn rotator cuff (partial)

INDICATIONS

- painful, limited ROM of the shoulder
- loss of strength with overhead activity

ALTERNATIVE TREATMENTS

- continued nonoperative management
- corticosteroid injections
- arthroscopic repair

SURGICAL ANATOMY

Incisions
Saber, or mini-open after arthroscopic acromioplasty

APPROACHES

Surgical Techniques
- Saber incision or mini-open after arthroscopic acromioplasty
- split or detach deltoid
- identify and release coracoacromial ligament
- ¾ inch osteotome to remove acromial spur
- rasp bone smooth
- identify torn cuff, perform rotator interval or capsular release as necessary to mobilize cuff
- reattach cuff through bone tunnels, use suture anchors or other fixation devices
- reattach deltoid with sutures through bone
- skin closure

POSTOPERATIVE MANAGEMENT

- sling for 6 weeks

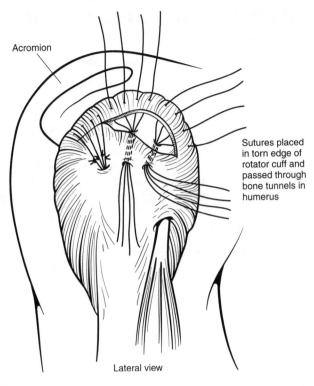

Acromion

Sutures placed
in torn edge of
rotator cuff and
passed through
bone tunnels in
humerus

Lateral view

REHABILITATION

- supine active-assisted forward elevation for 4–6 weeks
- rotator cuff strengthening at 6–8 weeks

COMPLICATIONS

- re-tear, continued pain
- capsulitis, loss of motion

SELECTED REFERENCES

Neer CS II. Anterior acromioplasty for the chronic impingement syndrome in the shoulder. J Bone Joint Surg Am 1972;54:41–50.

Bach BR. Multi-suture technique for open rotator cuff repair. Tech Shoulder Elbow Surg 2001;2(2):106–117.

TENODESIS, LONG TENDON OF BICEPS

CPT code   **23430** tenodesis of the long tendon of biceps

ICD-9 code   **726.12** biceps tenosynovitis

                      727.62 partial or complete tear of proximal biceps tendon

INDICATIONS

Pain, weakness, and limitation of motion due to chronic biceps tendonitis; recurrent subluxation of the biceps tendon; or rupture of the proximal biceps tendon that does not respond to rehabilitation, NSAIDs, or steroid injections.

ALTERNATIVE TREATMENTS

- continued nonoperative management
- tenotomy
- arthroscopic tenodesis

Incision
- deltopectoral

APPROACHES

Surgical Techniques
- deltopectoral approach
- identify bicipital groove
- open tendon sheath, place traction suture into biceps tendon
- deliver as much tendon from intra-articular space as possible and transect the tendon (note: tenotomy can be performed arthroscopically; when doing so, arthroscopically place a retention suture into the tendon prior to tenotomy)
- debride bicipital groove to bleeding bone
- tenodesis can be performed with one or two suture anchors, or
- using a motorized burr, create a "keyhole" into the tenodesis site
- roll the tendon into a ball and suture to maintain shape
- insert ball into keyhole and extend elbow

POSTOPERATIVE MANAGEMENT

- sling for comfort

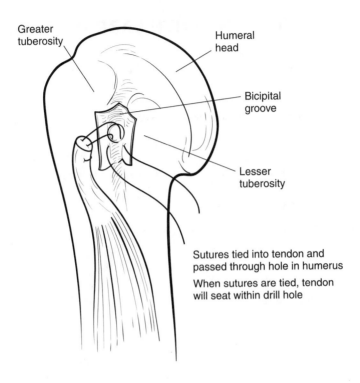

Greater tuberosity

Humeral head

Bicipital groove

Lesser tuberosity

Sutures tied into tendon and passed through hole in humerus

When sutures are tied, tendon will seat within drill hole

REHABILITATION

- active-assisted and passive motion, immediately
- strengthening for 4–6 weeks
- return to sport after 6–12 weeks

SELECTED REFERENCES

Berlman U, Bayley I. Tenodesis of the long head of biceps brachii in the painful shoulder: improving results in the long term. J Shoulder Elbow Surg 1995;4: 429–435.

Becker DA, Cofield RH. Tenodesis of the long head of the biceps brachii for chronic bicipital tendonitis. J Bone Joint Surg Am 1989;71:376–381.

NOTES

_____

_____

_____

_____

_____

CAPSULORRHAPHY WITH LABRAL REPAIR

CPT code	**23455** capsulorrhaphy with labral repair (e.g., Bankart repair)
ICD-9 codes	**718.31** recurrent dislocation of shoulder
	718.81 recurrent instability of the shoulder

INDICATIONS

Recurrent anterior instability, not responsive to strengthening program.

ALTERNATIVE TREATMENT

- arthroscopic Bankart repair, capsulorrhaphy

SURGICAL ANATOMY

Incision

- anterior deltopectoral

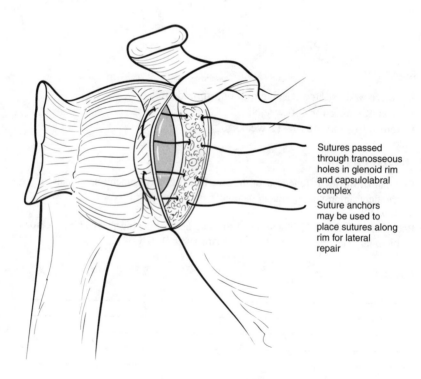

Sutures passed through tranosseous holes in glenoid rim and capsulolabral complex

Suture anchors may be used to place sutures along rim for lateral repair

APPROACHES

Surgical Techniques

- anterior skin incision from axilla to coracoid
- identify and protect cephalic vein
- incise clavipectoral fascia to coracoid, beware of musculocutaneous nerve
- incise or split subscapularis muscle and tag
- perform anterior capsulotomy
- repair Bankart lesion to bone with suture and anchors or with transosseous holes
- perform capsulorrhaphy
- reattach subscapularis with no. 2 permanent suture

POSTOPERATIVE MANAGEMENT

- sling for 2–4 weeks

REHABILITATION

- active-assisted and passive motion
- rotator cuff strengthening, and reestablish range of motion at 6 weeks
- return to sport at 5–6 months

COMPLICATIONS

- recurrent instability
- loss of motion
- hardware problems
- axillary nerve, musculocutaneous nerve injury

SELECTED REFERENCES

Levine WN, Richmond JC, Donaldson WR. Use of the suture anchor in open Bankart reconstruction. A follow-up report. Am J Sports Med 1994;22(5):723–726.

Cole BJ, L'Insalata J, Irrgang J, Warner JJ. Comparison of arthroscopic and open anterior shoulder stabilization. A two-six year follow-up study. J Bone Joint Surg Am 2000;82A:1108–1114.

NOTES

_____

_____

_____

_____

_____

CAPSULORRHAPHY, ANTERIOR, WITH CORACOID PROCESS TRANSFER

CPT code   23462 capsulorrhaphy, anterior, with coracoid process transfer (Bristow procedure, Bristow-Latarjet procedure)

ICD-9 codes   718.31 recurrent dislocation of the shoulder
             728.41 laxity of shoulder ligaments

INDICATIONS

Recurrent anterior dislocations or subluxations of the glenohumeral joint, not responsive to activity modification and physical therapy that includes shoulder strengthening for a period of at least 3 months.

ALTERNATIVE TREATMENTS

- open Bankart repair
- arthroscopic Bankart repair
- open anterior capsular shift
- arthroscopic capsulorrhaphy

SURGICAL ANATOMY

Incision
- deltopectoral incision
- anterior axillary line incision

APPROACHES

Surgical Techniques
- supine position, roll under scapula
- deltopectoral approach, cephalic vein lateral
- identify coracoid process medial to coracobrachialis
- drill 2.5-mm hole in coracoid tip, osteotomize coracoid
- incise subscapularis tendon vertically
- split subscapularis and capsule transversely
- drill hole in anterior-inferior glenoid, attach coracoid with AO screw (4.5 malleolar screw)
- reattach subscapularis tendon (inferior flap under conjoined tendon)
- layered closure

POSTOPERATIVE MANAGEMENT

- sling and swathe for 4 weeks

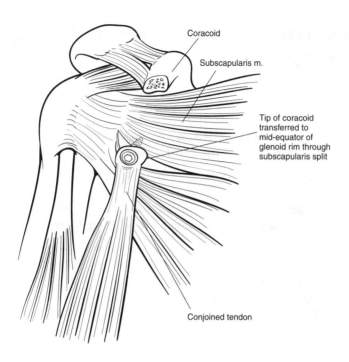

Coracoid

Subscapularis m.

Tip of coracoid
transferred to
mid-equator of
glenoid rim through
subscapularis split

Conjoined tendon

REHABILITATION

- active–assisted ROM for 4 weeks
- strengthening for 6 weeks
- sports at 3 months
- contact sports at 6 months

COMPLICATIONS

- recurrent subluxation
- hardware migration
- non-union of coracoid transfer
- intra-articular violation with screw; arthrosis

SELECTED REFERENCES

May VR Jr. A modified Bristow operation for anterior recurrent dislocation of the shoulder. J Bone Joint Surg Am 1970;52:1010–1016.
Hovelius LK, Sandstrom BC, Rosmark DL, et al. Long-term results with the Bankart and Bristow procedures. J Shoulder Elbow Surg 2001;10:445–452.

CAPSULORRHAPHY, GLENOHUMERAL JOINT, POSTERIOR

CPT code   23465 capsulorrhaphy, glenohumeral joint, posterior, with or without bone block

ICD-9 codes   718.31 recurrent dislocations of the shoulder
                  718.81 recurrent instability of the shoulder

INDICATIONS

Recurrent posterior dislocations or subluxations of the shoulder not responsive to physical therapy, including strengthening for at least 3 months.

ALTERNATIVE TREATMENTS

- open posterior shift/infraspinatus tenodesis
- arthroscopic posterior capsular shift
- shoulder fusion

SURGICAL ANATOMY

Incision

- horizontal incision 1 cm inferior to scapular spine, or
- vertical incision from acromion to axillary crease

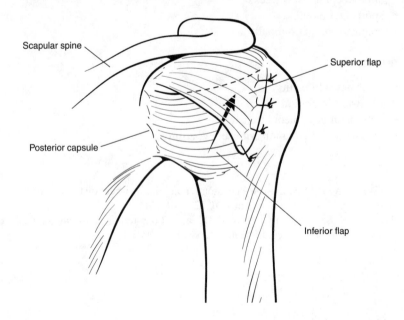

Scapular spine

Superior flap

Posterior capsule

Inferior flap

APPROACHES

Surgical Techniques

- lateral decubitus position
- surgical incision
- split or detach deltoid muscle
- detach infraspinatus tendon ¼ inch from tuberosity
- can also split between infraspinatus and teres muscle
- dissect infraspinatus tendon from capsule
- transverse capsulotomy
- repair any labral avulsions with suture anchors
- detach capsule vertically, 1 cm medial to humeral insertion to 6 o'clock inferiorly; leave teres minor tendon attached (note: capsule may be shifted on glenoid—see Fronek et al)
- shift inferior flap superiorly
- reattach flap to capsular stump with arm in 20–30° of external rotation
- reattach infraspinatus tendon
- layered closure

POSTOPERATIVE MANAGEMENT

- immobilized in 10° of external rotation for 6 weeks

REHABILITATION

- assisted motion at 6 weeks
- strengthening at 3 months
- return to sport with FROM and strength for 4–6 months

COMPLICATIONS

- recurrent instability
- axillary nerve injury

SELECTED REFERENCES

Neer CS II, Foster CR. Inferior capsular shift for instability of the shoulder. J Bone Joint Surg Am 1980;62:897–908.

Fronek J, Warren RF, Bowen M. Posterior subluxation of the glenohumeral joint. J Bone Joint Surg Am 1989;71:205–216.

CAPSULORRHAPHY, GLENOHUMERAL JOINT, ANY INSTABILITY

CPT code   **23466** capsulorrhaphy, multi-directional, any type

ICD-9 codes   **718.31** recurrent dislocation of the shoulder
                      718.81 recurrent instability of the shoulder
                      728.41 laxity of shoulder ligaments

INDICATIONS

Recurrent dislocations, subluxations, and/or pain of the shoulder associated with a sulcus sign, not responsive to activity modification and physical therapy that includes shoulder strengthening for a period of at least 3–6 months.

ALTERNATIVE TREATMENTS

- continued physical therapy
- arthroscopic capsulorraphy
- shoulder fusion

SURGICAL ANATOMY

Incisions

- deltopectoral incision or
- anterior axillary line incision

APPROACHES

Surgical Techniques

- supine position, roll under scapula
- deltopectoral approach, lateral to cephalic vein
- incise clavipectoral fascia, retract conjoined tendon medially
- identify axillary nerve
- incise subscapularis tendon, develop plane above capsule
- close rotator interval with shoulder externally rotated
- transverse capsulotomy and examine for Bankart lesion
- develop upper and lower capsular flaps
- place no. 2 sutures in capsular tags on humerus
- tension inferior flap superiorly and suture to humerus using previously placed sutures—suture anchors may also be used
- tension inferior flap and suture over superior flap
- reattach subscapularis tendon
- layered closure

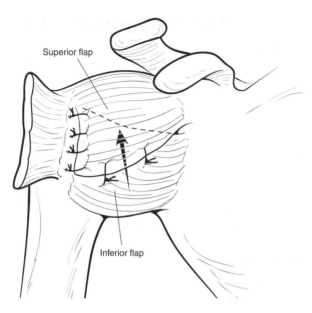

POSTOPERATIVE MANAGEMENT

- sling and swathe—4 weeks

REHABILITATION

- active-assisted ROM
- strengthening for 6 weeks
- sports at 3 months
- contact sports at 6 months

COMPLICATIONS

- recurrent instability, pain
- axillary nerve injury, loss of motion

SELECTED REFERENCES

Schenk TJ, Brems JJ. Multidirectional instability of the shoulder. J Am Acad Orthop Surg 1998;6:65–72.

Neer CS II, Foster CR. Inferior capsular shift for involuntary inferior and multidirectional instability of the shoulder. J Bone Joint Surg Am 1980;62:897–908.

OPEN TREATMENT OF ACROMIOCLAVICULAR DISLOCATION

CPT code   23550 open treatment of acromioclavicular dislocation, acute or chronic

ICD-9 code   831.04 acute/chronic acromioclavicular joint dislocation

INDICATIONS

acute and chronic: Type III dislocation and Type IV, V, VI dislocations
- pain at acromioclavicular (AC) joint region interfering with activity, sports
- failure of rehabilitation and injections to relieve symptoms

ALTERNATIVE TREATMENT

- sling for comfort, rehabilitation

SURGICAL ANATOMY

Incision
- anterosuperior Saber-type incision
- horizontal incision across anterior acromion and AC joint extending medially

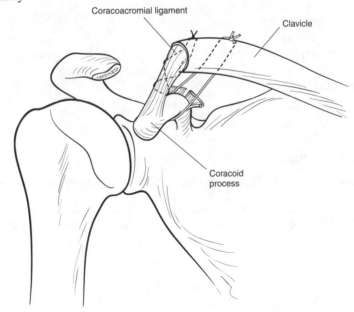

Coracoacromial ligament

Clavicle

Coracoid process

APPROACHES

Surgical Techniques

- create skin flaps
- incise, reflect anterior deltoid muscle
- incise deltotrapezial fascia and expose distal clavicle
- preserve, dissect coracoacromial ligament
- debride intra-articular meniscus
- reduce distal clavicle (other option is to resect distal 1.0–1.5 cm of distal clavicle)
- maintain reduction with transarticular K-wires; heavy nonabsorbable suture passed around base of clavicle and through drill hole in distal clavicle; or screw fixation from distal clavicle into base of coracoid
- transfer coracoacromial ligament into distal end of clavicle with drill holes and permanent suture
- repair deltoid to bone and reapproximate deltotrapezial fascia
- skin closure

POSTOPERATIVE MANAGEMENT

- sling for 6 weeks

REHABILITATION

- active-assisted and passive motion at 4–6 weeks
- rotator cuff strengthening
- return to sport in 12–16 weeks

COMPLICATIONS

- recurrent deformity
- pain, instability of distal clavicle

SELECTED REFERENCES

Nuber GW, Bowen MK. Acromioclavicular joint injuries and distal clavicle fractures. J Am Acad Orthop Surg 1997;5:11–18.
Guy DK, Wirth MA, Griffin JL, Rockwood CA. Reconstruction of chronic and complete dislocations of the acromioclavicular joint. Clin Orthop 1998;347:138–149.

NOTES

_____

_____

_____

_____

_____

OPEN TREATMENT OF ACROMIOCLAVICULAR DISLOCATION, WITH GRAFT

CPT code 23552 open treatment of acromioclavicular dislocation, acute or chronic with graft

ICD-9 code(s) 831.04 chronic acromioclavicular joint dislocation

INDICATIONS

Complete or unreduced dislocations of the AC joint (Type III dislocation; Type IV, V, VI dislocations)
- pain at AC joint region interfering with activity and sports
- failure of rehabilitation, injections to relieve symptoms

ALTERNATIVE TREATMENT

- sling for comfort, rehabilitation

SURGICAL ANATOMY

Incision
- anterosuperior Saber-type incision
- horizontal incision across anterior acromion and AC joint extending medially

APPROACHES

Surgical Techniques
- create skin flaps
- incise, reflect anterior deltoid muscle
- incise deltotrapezial fascia and expose distal clavicle
- debride intra-articular meniscus
- reduce distal clavicle (other option is to resect distal 1.0–1.5 cm of distal clavicle)
- maintain reduction with transarticular K-wires; heavy nonabsorbable suture passed around base of clavicle and through drill hole in distal clavicle; or screw fixation from distal clavicle into base of coracoid
- drill hole in distal clavicle junction, anterior mid-third
- pass graft (fascia lata, semitendinosus, allograft) through drill hole and around base of coracoid, suture together (may use suture anchors)
- repair deltoid to bone and reapproximate deltotrapezial fascia
- skin closure

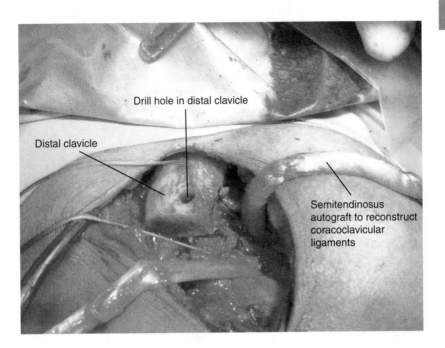

Drill hole in distal clavicle

Distal clavicle

Semitendinosus autograft to reconstruct coracoclavicular ligaments

POSTOPERATIVE MANAGEMENT

- sling for 6 weeks; protect against distal traction on arm keeping AC joint reduced

REHABILITATION

- active-assisted and passive motion at 4–6 weeks
- rotator cuff strengthening
- return to sport at 12–16 weeks

COMPLICATIONS

- recurrent deformity
- pain, instability of distal clavicle

SELECTED REFERENCES

Jones HP, Lemos MJ, Schepsis AA. Salvage of failed acromioclavicular joint reconstruction using autogenous semitendinosus tendon from the knee. Am J Sports Med 2001;29:234–237.

Guy DK, Wirth MA, Griffin JL, Rockwood CA. Reconstruction of chronic and complete dislocations of the acromioclavicular joint. Clin Orthop 1998;347:138–149.

SHOULDER ARTHROSCOPY, DIAGNOSTIC

CPT code   29805 shoulder arthroscopy—diagnostic

ICD-9 codes   718.81 derangement of shoulder joint
                 719.91 unspecified disorder of shoulder joint

INDICATIONS

Persistent pain, crepitus, feelings of instability not relieved by rest, NSAIDs, and rehabilitation, and for which other diagnostic tests have not identified the cause of the derangement.

ALTERNATIVE TREATMENTS

- arthrotomy
- magnetic resonance imaging (MRI)
- computed tomographic (CT) scan with contrast

SURGICAL ANATOMY

Incision

- posterior shoulder arthroscopy portal
- accessory portals: anterior-superior and anterior-inferior

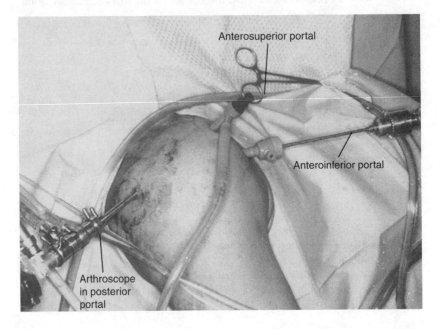

Anterosuperior portal

Anteroinferior portal

Arthroscope
in posterior
portal

APPROACHES

Surgical Techniques

- lateral decubitus or beach chair position
- mark cutaneous landmarks
- examination under anesthesia for ROM and anterior, inferior, and posterior laxity
- insert arthroscope into posterior portal
- systematic examination of joint including biceps tendon; superior labrum; superior, middle, and inferior glenohumeral ligaments; labrum; subscapularis tendon; inferior pouch; rotator cuff; and humeral and glenoid articular cartilage
- address pathologic condition identified

POSTOPERATIVE MANAGEMENT

- sling for comfort

REHABILITATION

- pendulum and Codman-type exercises
- specific rehabilitation depends on other procedures involved

COMPLICATIONS

- infection
- fluid extravasation
- neurovascular injury

SELECTED REFERENCES

Andrews JR, Carson WG Jr, Ortega K. Arthroscopy of the shoulder: techniques and normal anatomy. Am J Sports Med 1984;12:1–7.

Andrews JR, Heckman MM, Guerra JJ. Diagnostic arthroscopy of the shoulder. In: JB McGinty, RB Caspari, eds Operative arthroscopy, 2nd ed. Philadelphia: Lippincott-Raven, 1996.

NOTES

ARTHROSCOPIC CAPSULORRHAPHY, ANTERIOR

CPT code   **29806** arthroscopic capsulorrhaphy—anterior

ICD-9 codes   **718.31** recurrent dislocation of the shoulder
              718.81 instability of the shoulder

INDICATIONS

Recurrent dislocation, subluxation, or pain secondary to shoulder instability (without a Bankart lesion) that has not responded to a program of rehabilitation.

ALTERNATIVE TREATMENTS

- open anterior-inferior capsular shift
- arthroscopic transglenoid capsulorrhaphy
- arthroscopic thermal capsulorraphy
- shoulder fusion

SURGICAL ANATOMY

Incision
- beach chair or lateral decubitus position
- posterior portal
- accessory anterior-superior and anterior-inferior portals

APPROACHES

Surgical Techniques
- position patient
- examination under anesthesia
- insert arthroscope, diagnostic examination
- abrade anterior and inferior capsule using motorized shaver or rasp
- sequential "tucks" are made in capsule, 1 cm lateral to labrum and transferred with suture hook through labrum with PDS suture or suture shuttle relay device
- rotator interval closure

POSTOPERATIVE MANAGEMENT

- sling immobilization

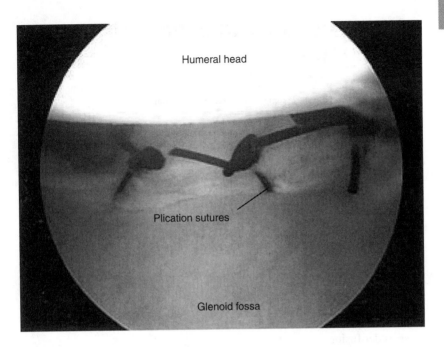

Humeral head

Plication sutures

Glenoid fossa

REHABILITATION

- sling immobilization for 4 weeks
- daily pendulum exercises
- physical therapy for ROM and strength
- return to noncontact sports with full ROM and strength
- avoid contact sports for 4–6 months

COMPLICATIONS

- recurrent instability
- infection
- axillary nerve injury

SELECTED REFERENCES

Nelson BJ, Arciero RA. Arthroscopic management of glenohumeral instability. Am J
    Sports Med 2000;28:602–614.
Tauro JC, Carter FM. Arthroscopic capsular advancement for anterior and anterior-
    inferior shoulder instability. Arthroscopy 1994;10:513–517.

ARTHROSCOPIC CAPSULORRHAPHY, POSTERIOR

CPT code   **29806** arthroscopic capsulorraphy—posterior

ICD-9 codes   **718.31** recurrent dislocation of the shoulder
                  718.81 instability of the shoulder

INDICATIONS

Recurrent dislocation, subluxation, or pain secondary to shoulder instability (without a Bankart lesion) that has not responded to a program of rehabilitation.

ALTERNATIVE TREATMENTS

- open posterior-inferior capsular shift
- arthroscopic transglenoid capsulorrhaphy
- arthroscopic thermal capsulorraphy
- shoulder fusion

SURGICAL ANATOMY

Incision
- beach chair or lateral decubitus position
- posterior portal; accessory posterior portal
- accessory anterior-superior portal

APPROACHES

Surgical Techniques
- position patient
- examination under anesthesia
- insert arthroscope, diagnostic examination
- abrade posterior and inferior capsule—CAUTION, capsule is thin—using motorized shaver or rasp
- abrade labrum
- sequential "tucks" are made in capsule, 1 cm lateral to labrum, and transferred with suture hook through labrum with PDS suture beginning inferior and continuing superior
- rotator interval closure

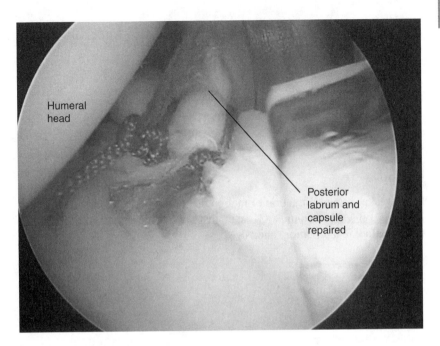

POSTOPERATIVE MANAGEMENT

- sling immobilization for 4–6 weeks

REHABILITATION

- sling immobilization for 4 weeks
- daily pendulum exercises
- physical therapy for ROM and strength
- return to noncontact sports with full ROM and strength
- avoid contact sports for 4–6 months

COMPLICATIONS

- recurrent instability
- infection
- axillary nerve injury

SELECTED REFERENCES

Nelson BJ, Arciero RA. Arthroscopic management of glenohumeral instability. Am J Sports Med 2000;28:602–614.

Antoniou J, Duckworth DT, Harryman DT 2nd. Capsulolabral augmentation for the management of posteroinferior instability of the shoulder. J Bone Joint Surg Am 2000;8:1220–1230.

ARTHROSCOPIC REPAIR OF SLAP LESION, SUTURE ANCHOR TECHNIQUE

CPT code   29807 arthroscopic repair of superior labrum anterior to posterior (SLAP) lesion (suture anchor technique)

ICD-9 code(s)   840.7 labral tear, shoulder

INDICATIONS

Pain, weakness, and limitation of motion due to a superior labral tear, identified on MRI or contrast CT scan, that does not improve with activity modification, rehabilitation, and NSAIDs.

ALTERNATIVE TREATMENTS

- activity modification
- open labral repair

SURGICAL ANATOMY

Incision
- anterior direct lateral (see Selected References) and posterior portal

APPROACHES

Surgical Techniques
- insert arthroscope posteriorly
- establish anterior portal through rotator interval
- evaluate glenohumeral joint
- identify superior labral tear
- debride superior glenoid tubercle to bleeding bone through anterior portal
- establish lateral portal through rotator cuff
- drill and insert suture anchor through lateral portal according to manufacturer's instructions (note: a variety of devices, including knotless anchors, are available)
- shuttle one limb of suture through superior labrum and out anterior portal (note: a variety of devices are available)
- grasp anterior suture and bring back into lateral portal
- tie knot to secure labrum
- repeat every 8–10 mm of detached labrum, if necessary

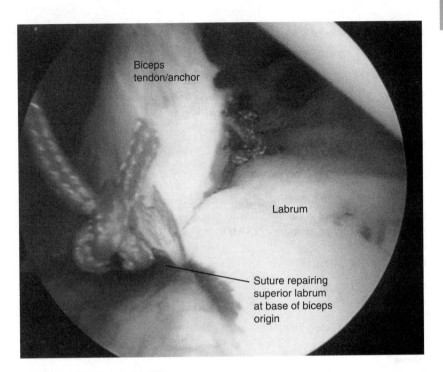

POSTOPERATIVE MANAGEMENT

- sling for 2–3 weeks

REHABILITATION

- active-assisted and active ROM at 3 weeks
- rotator cuff strengthening for 4–6 weeks
- return to sport after 12–16 weeks

COMPLICATIONS

- recurrent pain, inability to return to sport or work
- infection, hardware/anchor impingement or migration

SELECTED REFERENCES

Snyder SJ, Karzel RP, Del Pizzo W, et al. SLAP lesions of the shoulder. Arthroscopy
     1990;6:274–279.
Snyder SJ, Banas MP, Karzel RP. An analysis of 140 injuries to the superior glenoid
     labrum. J Shoulder Elbow Surg 1995;4:243–248.

ARTHROSCOPIC REPAIR OF SLAP LESION, ARTHROSCOPIC TACK TECHNIQUE

CPT code   29807 arthroscopic repair of superior labrum anterior to posterior (SLAP) lesion (arthroscopic tack technique)

ICD-9 code   840.7 labral tear, shoulder

INDICATIONS

Pain, weakness, and limitation of motion due to superior labral tear identified on MRI or contrast CT scan that does not improve with activity modification, rehabilitation, or NSAIDs.

ALTERNATIVE TREATMENTS

- activity modification
- open labral repair

SURGICAL ANATOMY

Incision
- anterior, direct lateral (see Selected References) and posterior portals

APPROACHES

Surgical Techniques
- insert arthroscope posteriorly, establish anterior portal through rotator interval
- complete glenohumeral evaluation
- identify superior labral avulsion
- debride superior glenoid tubercle to bleeding bone
- establish lateral portal
- using manufacturer's drill guide in the lateral portal, drill guide wire through labrum and into superior glenoid
- over-drill guide wire with cannulated drill bit, remove drill bit, guide wire remains in bone
- insert cannulated tack over guide wire and impact into glenoid to secure labrum to bone
- repeat every 8–10 mm of avulsed labrum, as necessary

POSTOPERATIVE MANAGEMENT

- sling for 2–3 weeks

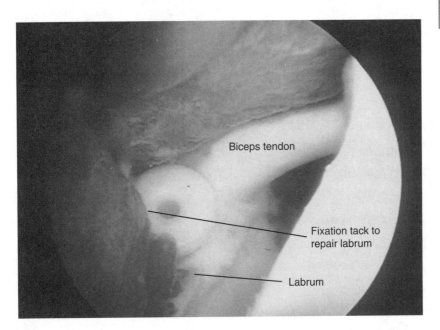

Biceps tendon

Fixation tack to repair labrum

Labrum

REHABILITATION

- active-assisted and passive motion for 3 weeks
- rotator cuff strengthening for 4–6 weeks
- return to sport after 12–16 weeks

COMPLICATIONS

- recurrent pain
- recurrent tear

SELECTED REFERENCES

Pagnani MJ, Speer KP, Altchek DW, et al. Arthroscopic fixation of superior labral lesions using a biodegradable implant. Arthroscopy 1995;11:194–198.

Samani C, Marston SB, Buss DD. Arthroscopic stabilization of type II SLAP lesions using an absorbable tack. Arthroscopy 2001;17:119–124.

NOTES

ARTHROSCOPY, FOREIGN BODY REMOVAL

CPT code   29819 removal of loose body

ICD-9 codes   718.81 derangement of shoulder joint
                  719.91 unspecified disorder of shoulder joint

INDICATIONS

- pain, crepitus, and mechanical symptoms not responsive to nonoperative treatment

ALTERNATIVE TREATMENTS

- arthrotomy
- MRI
- CT scan with contrast

SURGICAL ANATOMY

Incision
- posterior shoulder arthroscopy, portal
- accessory portals, anterior-superior and anterior-inferior

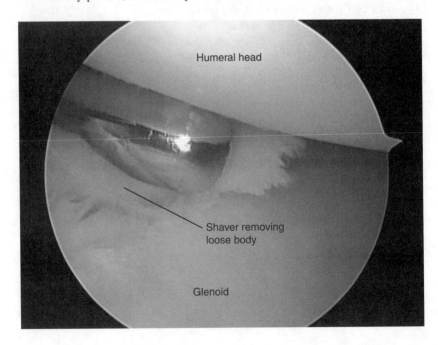

Humeral head

Shaver removing loose body

Glenoid

APPROACHES

Surgical Techniques
- lateral decubitus or beach chair position
- mark cutaneous landmarks
- examination under anesthesia for ROM and anterior, inferior, and posterior laxity
- insert arthroscope into posterior portal
- systematic examination of joint including biceps tendon; superior labrum; superior, middle, and inferior glenohumeral ligaments; labrum; subscapularis tendon; inferior pouch; rotator cuff; and humeral and glenoid articular cartilage
- address pathologic conditions identified
- use grasping instruments to remove loose bodies

POSTOPERATIVE MANAGEMENT

- sling for comfort

REHABILITATION

- pendulum and Codman-type exercises
- specific rehabilitation depends on other procedures involved

COMPLICATIONS

- infection
- fluid extravasation
- neurovascular injury

SELECTED REFERENCES

Andrews JR, Carson WG Jr, Ortega K. Arthroscopy of the shoulder: techniques and normal anatomy. Am J Sports Med 1984;12:1–7.
Andrews JR, Heckman MM, Guerra JJ. Diagnostic arthroscopy of the shoulder. In: JB McGinty, RB Caspari, eds. Operative arthroscopy, 2nd ed. Philadelphia: Lippincott-Raven, 1996.

NOTES

_____
_____
_____
_____
_____
_____

ARTHROSCOPIC SYNOVECTOMY

CPT code   29820/29821 arthroscopic synovectomy
                  29820 partial, 29821 complete

ICD-9 codes   213.7 synovial chrondromatosis
                  711.01 septic arthritis
                  714.0 rheumatoid arthritis
                  719.21 pigmented villonodular synovitis

INDICATIONS

Pain and limitation of motion due to synovial diseases (rheumatoid arthritis [RA], pigmented villonodular synovitis [PVNS], synovial chondromatosis, or septic arthritis [SA]) that have failed to respond to appropriate medical management.

ALTERNATIVE TREATMENTS

- medical therapy, RA
- intra-articular injections, RA
- serial aspirations, SA
- arthrotomy and open debridement

SURGICAL ANATOMY

Incision
- anterior and posterior portals

APPROACHES

- multiple loose bodies in axillary pouch (synovial osteochondromatosis)

Surgical Techniques
- insert arthroscope posteriorly
- establish anterior portal through rotator interval
- thoroughly irrigate the joint
- debride pathologic synovium with arthroscopic shaver (note: pathologic synovium will be found at the insertion of the rotator cuff into the humerus, and in the recesses anteriorly, superiorly over the glenoid labrum, and in the inferior pouch)
- remove loose bodies with arthroscopic grasping device

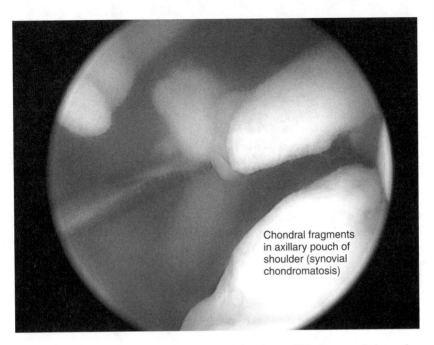

Chondral fragments in axillary pouch of shoulder (synovial chondromatosis)

- remove arthroscope, leaving sheath in joint, insert Wissinger rod through sheath and out anterior portal
- switch arthroscope to anterior portal
- repeat above process from posterior portal

POSTOPERATIVE MANAGEMENT

- sling for comfort

REHABILITATION

- active-assisted and passive motion, immediately
- rotator cuff strengthening for 4–6 weeks
- return to activity, variable

SELECTED REFERENCES

Bynum CK, Tasto J. Arthroscopic treatment of synovial disorders in the shoulder, elbow, and ankle. Am J Knee Surg 2002;15:57–59.

Matthews LS, LaBudde JF. Arthroscopic treatment of synovial diseases of the shoulder. Orthop Clin North Am 1993;24:101–109.

ARTHROSCOPIC RESECTION, DISTAL CLAVICLE, THREE PORTAL TECHNIQUE

CPT code   29824 arthroscopic resection of the distal clavicle (three portal technique)

ICD-9 codes   715.91 acromioclavicular arthritis

718.31 chronic dislocation

840.0 chronic acromioclavicular joint sprain, osteolysis

INDICATIONS

Pain and limitation of motion secondary to degeneration of the AC joint that does not respond to at least 3 months of rehabilitation, NSAIDs, and corticosteroid injections.

ALTERNATIVE TREATMENTS

- repeated injections of corticosteroid
- open resection of the distal clavicle (Mumford/Gurd procedure)

SURGICAL ANATOMY

Incision
- posterior, anterior, and lateral portals

APPROACHES

Surgical Techniques
- arthroscopic glenohumeral evaluation
- arthroscope into subacromial space (post)
- subtotal bursectomy through lateral portal (arthroscopic shaver or radiofrequency wand)
- acromioplasty (if indicated)
- arthroscope to lateral portal
- subperiosteal stripping of anterior, inferior, and posterior 1-cm distal clavicle (radiofrequency wand or shaver in anterior portal); may use posterior portal as well
- resect 1-cm distal clavicle through anterior portal with motorized burr

POSTOPERATIVE MANAGEMENT

- sling for comfort (cryotherapy)

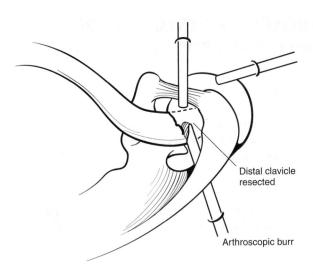

Distal clavicle
resected

Arthroscopic burr

REHABILITATION

- active-assisted and passive motion, day 1
- rotator cuff strengthening for 2–4 weeks
- return to sport after 6–12 weeks

COMPLICATIONS

- inadequate resection, continued pain
- infection
- aggressive resection, instability

SELECTED REFERENCES

Kay SP, Ellman H, Harris R. Arthroscopic distal clavicle excision: technique and
early results. Clin Orthop 1994;301:181–184.
Bell RH. Distal clavicle excision. Instr Course Lect 1998;47:35–41.

NOTES

ARTHROSCOPIC RESECTION, DISTAL CLAVICLE, TWO PORTAL TECHNIQUE

CPT code   29824 arthroscopic resection of the distal clavicle (two portal technique)

ICD-9 code(s)   715.91 chronic acromioclavicular arthritis

718.31 chronic acromioclavicular sprain

840.0 osteolysis

INDICATIONS

Pain and limitation of motion secondary to degeneration of the AC joint that does not respond to at least 3 months of rehabilitation, NSAIDs, and cortico-steroid injections.

ALTERNATIVE TREATMENTS

- repeated injections of corticosteroid
- open resection of the distal clavicle (Mumford/Gurd procedure)

SURGICAL ANATOMY

Incision

- portal directly posterior to AC joint, anterior portal

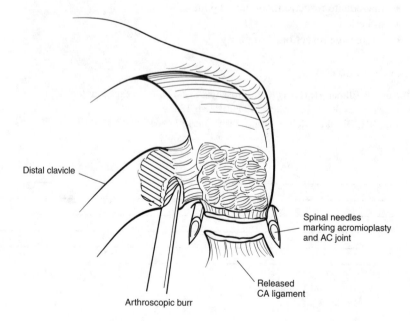

Distal clavicle

Spinal needles marking acromioplasty and AC joint

Released CA ligament

Arthroscopic burr

APPROACHES

Surgical Techniques

- arthroscopic glenohumeral evaluation
- arthroscope into subacromial space (post)
- radiofrequency wand or shaver to anterior portal
- subperiosteal stripping of anterior, inferior, and posterior 1-cm distal clavicle (radiofrequency wand or shaver in anterior portal)
- resect 1-cm distal clavicle through anterior portal
- can also be done through direct AC-joint approach:
  use 2.7 scope through posterior AC-joint portal to inspect joint and begin resection using a direct anterior AC-joint portal
  switch scope to anterior AC-joint portal and finish resection of posterior clavicle with burr in posterior AC-joint portal

POSTOPERATIVE MANAGEMENT

- sling for comfort (cryotherapy)

REHABILITATION

- active-assisted and passive motion, day 1
- rotator cuff strengthening for 2–4 weeks
- return to sport 6–12 weeks

COMPLICATIONS

- infection
- inadequate resection
- aggressive resection, instability

SELECTED REFERENCES

Levine WN, Barron OA, Yamaguchi K, et al. Arthroscopic distal clavicle resection through a bursal approach. Arthroscopy 1998;14:52–56.
Flatow EL, Cordasco FA, Bigliani LU. Arthroscopic resection of the outer end of the clavicle from a superior approach: a critical, quantitative, radiographic assessment of bone removal. Arthroscopy 1992;8:55–64.

NOTES

_____
_____
_____
_____
_____

ARTHROSCOPIC LYSIS AND RESECTION OF ADHESIONS

CPT code	29825 arthroscopic lysis and resection of adhesions with/without manipulation (Note: a variety of combinations of manipulation and capsular resection are published—please refer to Selected References.)
ICD-9 codes	718.41 contracture 726.0 adhesive capsulitis

INDICATIONS

Pain and limitation of motion due to either idiopathic or postsurgical adhesive capsulitis (frozen shoulder) that does not respond to at least 6 months of rehabilitation, NSAIDs, and possibly intra-articular steroid injections.

ALTERNATIVE TREATMENTS

- continued physical therapy
- closed manipulation under anesthesia
- open capsular contracture release

SURGICAL ANATOMY

Incision
- anterior and posterior portal

APPROACHES

Surgical Techniques
- insufflate joint with saline (to guard against injury to the articular cartilage during arthroscope insertion)
- establish anterior portal through rotator interval
- resect rotator interval tissue until full external rotation is restored (shaver, electrocautery, radiofrequency device)
- continue capsular release through middle and inferior glenohumeral ligaments
- remove instruments, manipulate
- if internal rotation is absent, release posterior superior capsule (scope anterior, wand posterior)
- if abduction/flexion absent, further release inferior pouch

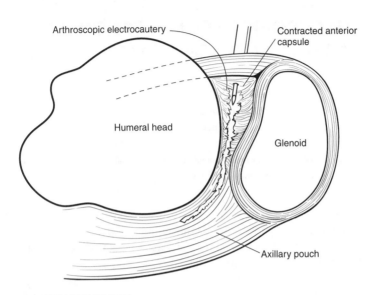

Arthroscopic electrocautery

Contracted anterior capsule

Humeral head

Glenoid

Axillary pouch

POSTOPERATIVE MANAGEMENT

- sling for comfort

REHABILITATION

- active-assisted and passive motion, immediately
- rotator cuff strengthening for 4 weeks
- return to sport after 6–12 weeks

COMPLICATIONS

- residual stiffness, loss of motion
- axillary nerve injury

SELECTED REFERENCES

Warner JJ. Frozen shoulder diagnosis and management. J Am Acad Orthop Surg 1997;5:130–140.
Bennett WF. Addressing glenohumeral stiffness while treating the painful and stiff shoulder arthroscopically. Arthroscopy 2000;16:142–150.

NOTES

_____

_____

_____

_____

_____

ARTHROSCOPIC DECOMPRESSION OF SUBACROMIAL SPACE, ELLMAN TECHNIQUE

CPT code   29826 arthroscopic decompression of the subacromial space with partial acromioplasty, with or without resection of the coracoacromial ligament (Ellman technique)

ICD-9 codes   726.10 chronic impingement (disorder of bursae and tendons, shoulder)
840.4 partial rotator cuff tear

INDICATIONS

Pain and limitation of motion due to subacromial impingement of the supraspinatus that does not respond to at least 3 months of rehabilitation, NSAIDs, and subacromial steroid injections.

ALTERNATIVE TREATMENTS

- continued physical therapy
- open acromioplasty

SURGICAL ANATOMY

Incision

- anterior, posterior, and lateral subacromial portals

APPROACHES

Surgical Techniques

- complete glenohumeral arthroscopy with examination of the rotator cuff, subscapularis tendon, and biceps tendon
- arthroscope to subacromial space, posterior portal
- shaver or radiofrequency wand to lateral portal
- subtotal bursectomy
- remove coracoacromial ligament from anterior acromion
- insert motorized acromionizer blade into lateral portal
- progressively remove anterior acromion from laterally to medially (see Illustration)

POSTOPERATIVE MANAGEMENT

- sling for comfort

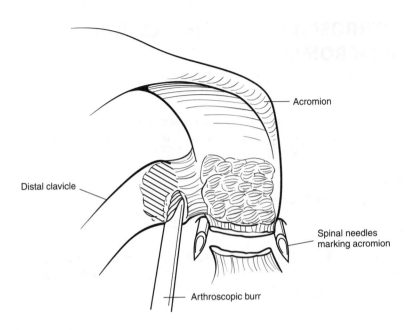

REHABILITATION

- active-assisted and passive motion
- rotator cuff strengthening
- return to sport after 6–12 weeks

COMPLICATIONS

- continued pain
- loss of motion
- proximal migration of humeral head if cuff tear present
- inadequate resection

SELECTED REFERENCES

Ellman H. Arthroscopic treatment of impingement of the shoulder. Instr Course Lect 1989;38:177–185.
Ellman H, Kay SP. Arthroscopic subacromial decompression for chronic impingement: two to five year results. J Bone Joint Surg Br 1991;73:395–398.

NOTES

ARTHROSCOPIC DECOMPRESSION OF SUBACROMIAL SPACE, CUTTING-BLOCK TECHNIQUE

CPT code   **29826** arthroscopic decompression of the subacromial space with partial acromioplasty, with or without resection of the coracoacromial ligament (cutting-block technique)

ICD-9 code(s)   **726.10** chronic impingement (disorder or bursae and tendons)
840.4 partial rotator cuff tear

INDICATIONS

Pain and limitation of motion due to subacromial impingement of the supraspinatus that does not respond to at least 3 months of rehabilitation, NSAIDs, and subacromial steroid injections.

ALTERNATIVE TREATMENTS

- continued physical therapy
- open acromioplasty

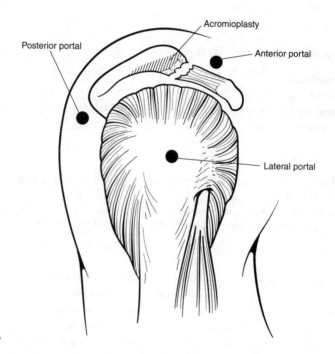

SURGICAL ANATOMY

Incision

- anterior, posterior, and lateral subacromial portals

APPROACHES

Surgical Techniques

- complete glenohumeral arthroscopy with examination of the rotator cuff, subscapularis tendon, and biceps tendon
- arthroscope to subacromial space-posterior portal
- shaver or radiofrequency wand to lateral portal
- subtotal bursectomy
- remove coracoacromial ligament from anterior acromion
- arthroscope to lateral portal
- arthroscopic acromionizer to posterior portal
- flatten with "cutting-block technique" (see illustration)

POSTOPERATIVE MANAGEMENT

- sling for comfort

REHABILITATION

- active-assisted and passive motion
- rotator cuff strengthening
- return to sport 6–12 weeks

COMPLICATIONS

- continued pain
- loss of motion
- proximal migration of humeral head if cuff tear present
- inadequate resection

SELECTED REFERENCE

Caspari RB, Thal R. A technique for arthroscopic subacromial decompression. Arthroscopy 1992;8:23–30.

NOTES

_____

_____

_____

_____

_____

ARTHROSCOPIC BANKART REPAIR AND CAPSULORRHAPHY FOR ANTERIOR INSTABILITY

CPT code   29806 unlisted code

29999 arthroscopic Bankart repair and capsulorrhaphy for anterior instability

ICD-9 codes   718.31 recurrent shoulder dislocation

718.91 instability of the shoulder joint

INDICATIONS

Recurrent dislocation, subluxation, or pain in the shoulder joint secondary to shoulder instability (with a Bankart lesion) that has not responded to a rehabilitation program.

ALTERNATIVE TREATMENT

- open Bankart repair and anterior-inferior capsular shift

SURGICAL ANATOMY

Incision
- posterior portal
- accessory anterior-superior and anterior-inferior portals

APPROACHES

Surgical Techniques
- patient in beach chair or lateral decubitus position
- examination under anesthesia
- arthroscope in posterior portal
- cannula in anterior portal; second cannula anterior-inferior portal
- elevate and mobilize Bankart lesion, decorticate glenoid
- grasp capsule and labrum and pass "0" PDS or shuttle relay, retrieve from anterosuperior portal
- place anchor on glenoid at 5 o'clock position for right shoulder; 7 o'clock for left
- use PDS or shuttle relay to shuttle nonabsorbable suture on anchor through tissue; tie arthroscopic knot
- repeat for two more anchors, proceeding proximally
- perform arthroscopic capsulorrhaphy as needed including posterior-inferior capsule

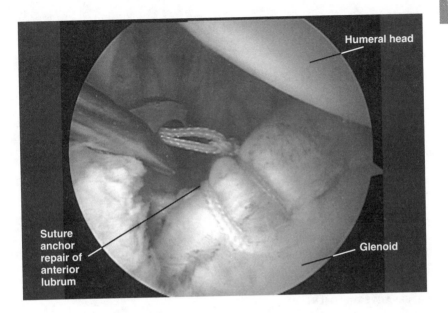

POSTOPERATIVE MANAGEMENT

- sling or sling and swathe for 3–4 weeks

REHABILITATION

- sling for 2–4 weeks
- initiate motion at 2 weeks
- strengthening at 4 weeks
- continue physical therapy exercises until full ROM and strength is achieved
- return to noncontact sports with full ROM and strength
- contact sports in 6 months

COMPLICATIONS

- recurrent instability
- axillary nerve injury
- anchor hardware impingement, migration problems

SELECTED REFERENCES

Cole BJ, Romeo AA. Arthroscopic shoulder stabilization with suture anchors: technique, technology, and pitfalls. Clin Orthop 2001;390:17–30.

Field M H, Field LD, Savoie FH. Arthroscopic labral repair with suture anchors. In: Warren, Craig, Altchek eds. The unstable shoulder. Philadelphia: Lippincott-Raven, 1999:315–328.

ARTHROSCOPIC BANKART REPAIR AND CAPSULORRHAPHY FOR POSTERIOR INSTABILITY

CPT code	29999 arthroscopic Bankart repair and capsulorrhaphy for posterior instability (unlisted code)
ICD-9 codes	718.31 recurrent shoulder dislocation
	718.91 instability of the shoulder joint

INDICATIONS

Recurrent dislocation, subluxation, or pain in the shoulder joint secondary to shoulder instability (with a Bankart lesion) that has not responded to rehabilitation.

ALTERNATIVE TREATMENT

- open posterior Bankart repair and posterior-inferior capsular shift

SURGICAL ANATOMY

Incision

- posterior portal, accessory posterior portal
- accessory anterior-superior portal

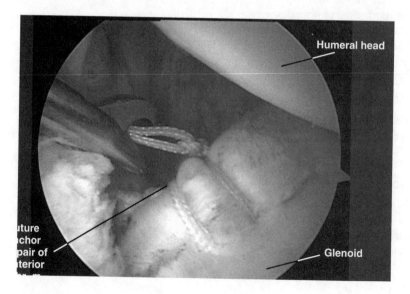

Humeral head

uture
chor
pair of
terior

Glenoid

APPROACHES

Surgical Techniques

- patient in beach chair or lateral decubitus position
- examination under anesthesia
- arthroscope in anterior-superior portal
- cannula in posterior portal; second cannula in posterior-inferior portal
- elevate and mobilize Bankart lesion, decorticate glenoid
- grasp capsule and labrum and pass '0' PDS or shuttle relay, retrieve from anterior-superior portal
- place anchor on glenoid at 7 o'clock position for right shoulder; 5 o'clock for left
- use PDS or shuttle relay to shuttle nonabsorbable suture on anchor through tissue; tie arthroscopic knot
- repeat for two more anchors proceeding proximally
- perform arthroscopic capsulorrhaphy as needed, including posterior-inferior capsule
- close rotator cuff interval

POSTOPERATIVE MANAGEMENT

- sling with arm in neutral rotation for 4 weeks

REHABILITATION

- sling for 2–4 weeks
- initiate motion at 2 weeks
- rotator cuff strengthening at 4 weeks
- continue physical therapy exercises until full ROM and strength is achieved
- return to noncontact sports with full ROM and strength
- contact sports in 6 months

COMPLICATIONS

- recurrent instability
- axillary nerve injury
- anchor hardware impingement, migration problems

SELECTED REFERENCES

Cole BJ, Romeo AA. Arthroscopic shoulder stabilization with suture anchors: technique, technology, and pitfalls. Clin Orthop 2001;390:17–30.

Antoniou J, Duckworth DT, Harryman DT 2nd. Capsulolabral augmentation for the management of posteroinferior instability of the shoulder. J Bone Joint Surg Am 2000;82:1220–1230.

ARTHROSCOPIC BANKART REPAIR AND CAPSULORRHAPHY FOR ANTERIOR INSTABILITY, TACK TECHNIQUE

CPT code	29999 arthroscopic Bankart repair and capsulorrhaphy for anterior instability, tack technique (unlisted code)
ICD-9 codes	718.31 recurrent shoulder dislocation
	718.91 instability of the shoulder joint

INDICATIONS

Recurrent dislocation, subluxation, or pain in the shoulder joint secondary to shoulder instability (with a Bankart lesion) that has not responded to rehabilitation.

ALTERNATIVE TREATMENTS

- open Bankart repair and anterior-inferior capsular shift
- arthroscopic Bankart with suture anchors

SURGICAL ANATOMY

Incisions
- posterior portal
- accessory anterior-superior and anterior-inferior portals

APPROACHES

Surgical Techniques
- patient in beach chair or lateral decubitus position
- examination under anesthesia
- arthroscope in posterior portal
- cannula in anterior portal; second cannula in anterior-inferior portal
- elevate and mobilize Bankart lesion, decorticate glenoid
- pierce capsule and labrum with guide wire-drill assembly and drill at 5 o'clock for right shoulder; 7 o'clock for left
- remove drill, leaving guide wire in place
- tap tack over guide wire into place securing lesion
- repeat for two more tacks, proceeding proximally
- perform arthroscopic capsulorrhaphy as needed, including posterior-inferior capsule with suture or radiofrequency energy

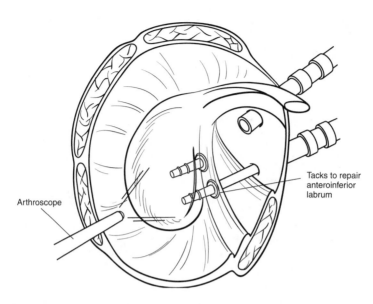

Arthroscope

Tacks to repair
anteroinferior
labrum

POSTOPERATIVE MANAGEMENT

- sling or sling and swathe, NO early motion

REHABILITATION

- sling for 2–4 weeks
- initiate motion at 2 weeks
- strengthening at 4 weeks
- continue physical therapy exercises until full ROM and strength is achieved
- return to noncontact sports with full ROM and strength
- contact sports in 6 months

COMPLICATIONS

- recurrent instability
- axillary nerve injury
- tack impingement, migration problems

SELECTED REFERENCES

Pagnani MJ, Dome DC. Surgical treatment of traumatic shoulder instability in American football players. J Bone Joint Surg Am 2002;84A:711–715.
Cole BJ, Romeo AA, Warner JJ. Arthroscopic Bankart repair with the Suretac device for traumatic anterior shoulder instability in athletes. Orthop Clin North Am 2001;32:411–421.

ARTHROSCOPIC THERMAL CAPSULORRHAPHY FOR POSTERIOR INSTABILITY

CPT code   **29999** arthroscopic thermal capsulorrhaphy for posterior instability
(unlisted code)

ICD-9 codes   **718.31** recurrent shoulder dislocation
718.91 instability of the shoulder joint

INDICATIONS

Recurrent posterior dislocation, subluxation, or pain in the shoulder joint secondary to shoulder instability (without a Bankart lesion) that has not responded to rehabilitation.

ALTERNATIVE TREATMENTS

- open posterior-inferior capsular shift
- arthroscopic posterior capsulorraphy
- shoulder fusion

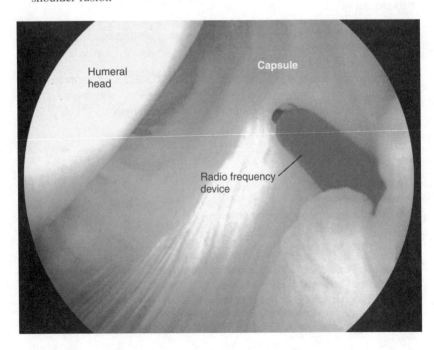

SURGICAL ANATOMY

Incision
- posterior portal
- accessory posterior-inferior portal
- anterior portal

APPROACHES

Surgical Techniques
- patient in beach chair or lateral decubitus position
- examination under anesthesia
- arthroscope in posterior portal
- cannula in anterior portal
- evaluate tissue—if thin, switch to a different method of stabilization
- apply thermal wand sequentially to tissues in pouch (turn power down at 5 o'clock and 7 o'clock to avoid axillary nerve)
- apply in rows, do not shrink entire capsule
- continue application to level of superior glenohumeral ligament

POSTOPERATIVE MANAGEMENT

- sling in neutral rotation, NO motion

REHABILITATION

- sling for 4 weeks
- initiate motion at 2 weeks
- strengthening at 4 weeks
- continue physical therapy exercises until full ROM and strength are achieved
- return to noncontact sports with full ROM and strength
- contact sports in 6 months

COMPLICATIONS

- recurrent instability
- axillary nerve injury
- ablation of capsule

SELECTED REFERENCES

Andrews JR, Dugas JR. Diagnosis and treatment of shoulder injuries in the throwing athlete: the role of thermal-assisted capsular shrinkage. AAOS Instr Course Lect 2001;50:17–21.

Hovis WD, Dean MT, Mallon WJ, Hawkins RJ. Posterior instability of the shoulder in elite golfers. Am J Sports Med 2002;30:886–890.

ARTHROSCOPIC THERMAL CAPSULORRHAPHY FOR ANTERIOR INSTABILITY

CPT code	29999	arthroscopic thermal capsulorrhaphy for anterior instability (unlisted code)

ICD-9 codes	718.31	recurrent shoulder dislocation
	718.91	instability of the shoulder joint

INDICATIONS

Recurrent dislocation, subluxation, or pain in the shoulder joint secondary to shoulder instability (without a Bankart lesion) that has not responded to rehabilitation.

ALTERNATIVE TREATMENTS

- open anterior-inferior capsular shift
- arthroscopic capsulorraphy
- shoulder fusion

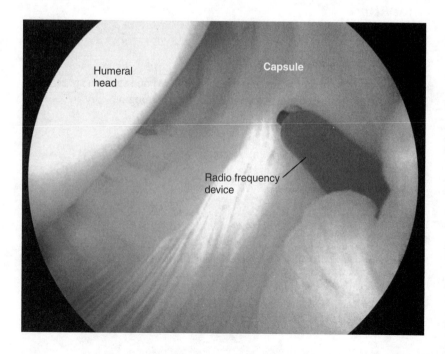

SURGICAL ANATOMY

Incisions

- posterior portal
- accessory anterior-superior and anterior-inferior portals

APPROACHES

Surgical Techniques

- patient in beach chair or lateral decubitus position
- examination under anesthesia
- arthroscope in posterior portal
- cannula in anterior portal
- evaluate tissue—if thin, switch to a different method of stabilization
- apply thermal wand sequentially to tissues in pouch (turn power down at 5 o'clock and 7 o'clock to avoid axillary nerve)
- apply in rows, do not shrink entire capsule
- continue application to level of superior glenohumeral ligament

POSTOPERATIVE MANAGEMENT

- sling or sling and swathe, NO early motion

REHABILITATION

- sling for 3–4 weeks
- begin motion at 4 weeks
- strengthening at 6 weeks
- continue physical therapy exercises until full ROM and strength is achieved
- return to noncontact sports with full ROM and strength
- contact sports in 6 months

COMPLICATIONS

- recurrent instability
- axillary nerve injury
- ablation of capsule

SELECTED REFERENCES

Andrews JR, Dugas JR. Diagnosis and treatment of shoulder injuries in the throwing athlete: the role of thermal-assisted capsular shrinkage. AAOS Instr Course Lect 2001;50:17–21.

Gerber A, Warner JJ. Thermal capsulorrhaphy to treat shoulder instability. Clin Orthop 2002;400:1105–1116.

ARTHROSCOPIC ROTATOR CUFF REPAIR

CPT code   29827 arthroscopic rotator cuff repair

ICD-9 code   727.61 torn rotator cuff (complete)
                    840.4 torn rotator cuff (partial)

INDICATIONS

Pain and loss of strength and motion, especially overhead.

ALTERNATIVE TREATMENTS

- continued rehabilitation
- corticosteroid injections
- open rotator cuff repair; mini-open repair

SURGICAL ANATOMY

Incision
- anterior and posterior portals

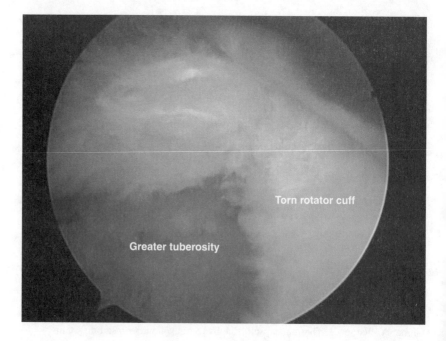

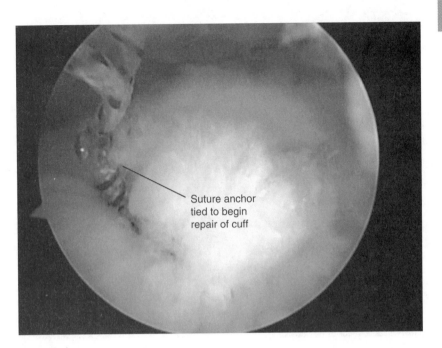

Suture anchor tied to begin repair of cuff

APPROACHES

Surgical Techniques

- glenohumeral arthroscopy
- identify cuff tear and configuration
- perform arthroscopic acromioplasty (CPT code 29826)
- abrade insertion area at greater tuberosity
- place two or three suture anchors posterior to anterior into greater tuberosity at "deadman's angle"
- using shuttle sutures or arthroscopic piercing/grasping instruments, pass sutures within anchors through torn edge of rotator cuff
- tie arthroscopic knots to secure repair

POSTOPERATIVE MANAGEMENT

- sling for 6 weeks

REHABILITATION

- supine active-assisted forward elevation for 4–6 weeks
- start to regain range of motion at 6 weeks
- rotator cuff strengthening at 6–8 weeks

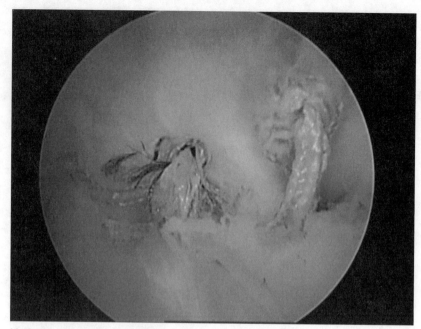

Multiple sutures used to repair tendon edge of supraspinatus

COMPLICATIONS

- re-tear, continued pain
- capsulitis, loss of motion

SELECTED REFERENCES

Yamaguchi K, Levine WN, Marra G, Galatz LM, Klepps S, Flatow E. Transitioning to arthroscopic rotator cuff repair: the pros and cons. J Bone Joint Surg Am 2003;85A:144–155.

Burkhart S. Arthroscopic repair of massive rotator cuff tear: concept of margin convergence. Tech Shoulder Elbow Surg 2000;1:240–246.

NOTES

_____

_____

_____

_____

_____

_____

_____

ARTHROSCOPIC ROTATOR INTERVAL CLOSURE

CPT code   29999 arthroscopic rotator interval closure (note: usually performed as an adjunctive procedure with arthroscopic procedures for instability)

ICD-9 code   see appropriate primary procedure

INDICATIONS

As an adjunct to arthroscopic instability procedures.

ALTERNATIVE TREATMENT

• see selected instability procedure

SURGICAL ANATOMY

Incision
• anterior and posterior portals

APPROACHES

Surgical Techniques
• perform all indicated primary procedures
• with arthroscope in posterior portal, pass absorbable suture through middle glenohumeral ligament from anterior portal (note: there are a variety of devices capable of passing suture in this manner)
• back anterior cannula out of joint to a level just superficial to the joint capsule
• pass an arthroscopic pointed grasping device through the capsule superior to the cannula insertion point (see Illustration) and use to grasp suture in joint and shuttle into cannula
• secure interval closure with a sliding knot
• procedure may be repeated to reinforce the interval closure
• remove cannula

POSTOPERATIVE MANAGEMENT

• as directed by primary procedure

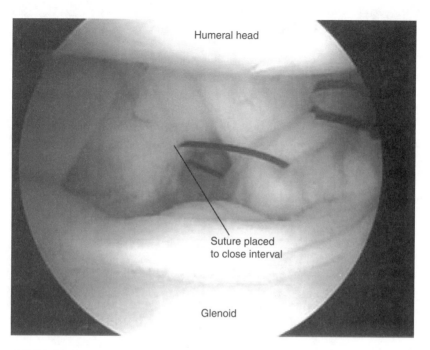

Humeral head

Suture placed
to close interval

Glenoid

REHABILITATION

- as directed by primary procedure

SELECTED REFERENCES

Gartsman GM, Taverna E, Hammerman SM. Arthroscopic rotator interval repair
  in glenohumeral instability. Arthroscopy 1999;15:330–332.
Treacy SH, Field LD, Savoie FH 3rd. Rotator interval capsule closure: an
  arthroscopic technique. Arthroscopy 1997;13:103–106.

NOTES

PART II

ELBOW

ARTHROTOMY, CAPSULAR RELEASE

CPT code   24006 arthrotomy, capsular release

ICD-9 code   718.42 contracture of elbow

INDICATIONS

- loss of elbow extension of greater than 30°
- failed rehabilitation, extension bracing

ALTERNATIVE TREATMENTS

- distraction arthrolysis
- arthroscopic release
- release of collateral ligaments, radial head resection

APPROACHES

Surgical Techniques

- proximal Kocher incision, 6 cm proximal to lateral epicondyle to 3 cm distal
- release extensor carpi radialis longus (ECRL) and brachioradialis from humerus
- elevate brachialis anteriorly, expose capsule
- excise lateral half of capsule, incise medial capsule
- if still loss of extension, elevate triceps from posterior humerus and release posterior capsule, resect soft tissue and osteophytes from olecranon fossa and olecranon

POSTOPERATIVE MANAGEMENT

- continuous passive motion (CPM), extension orthosis, splinting
- active and active-assisted range of motion (ROM)

COMPLICATIONS

- infection
- wound hematoma
- radial, ulnar, and medial nerve injury

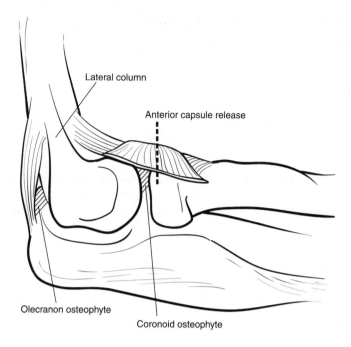

Lateral column

Anterior capsule release

Olecranon osteophyte

Coronoid osteophyte

REFERENCES

Husband JB, Hastings HH. The lateral approach for operative release of post-traumatic contracture of the elbow. J Bone Joint Surg Am 1990;72:1353–1358.
Mansat P, Morrey BF. The column procedure: a limited lateral approach for extrinsic contracture of the elbow. J Bone Joint Surg Am 1998;80:1603–1615.

NOTES

_____
_____
_____
_____
_____
_____
_____
_____

ARTHROTOMY OF ELBOW, LOOSE BODY REMOVAL

CPT code	24101 arthrotomy of elbow, loose body removal

ICD-9 code	718.12 loose body, elbow

INDICATIONS

Mechanical locking, catching, popping with elbow motion not relieved with rest, rehabilitation, NSAIDs. Positive imaging studies: radiographs, CT arthrography, or MRI.

ALTERNATIVE TREATMENT

* arthroscopic removal

APPROACHES

* supine
* prone
* lateral decubitus

Surgical Techniques

* lateral Kocher incision
* release proximally the ECRL and extensors to expose capsule
* incise capsule anteriorly and inspect, remove loose body
* reflect triceps posteriorly from humerus
* incise capsule posteriorly and inspect posterior joint

POSTOPERATIVE MANAGEMENT/REHABILITATION

* sling for comfort for 1–3 days and then motion
* passive ROM, active ROM, and progressive resistive exercise (PREs)

COMPLICATIONS

* infection
* wound hematoma
* radial nerve injury (with lateral approach)
* create posterolateral instability if lateral ulnar collateral ligament released

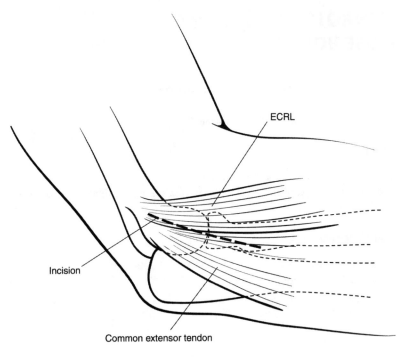

ECRL

Incision

Common extensor tendon

SELECTED REFERENCES

Crenshaw AH. Shoulder and elbow Injuries. In Crenshaw AH, ed. Campbell's operative orthopedics, 8th ed. Baltimore: CV Mosby, 1992:1741–1742.

Stother K, Day B, Regan WR. Arthroscopy of the elbow: anatomy, portal sites, and a description of the proximal lateral portal. Arthroscopy 1995:11:449–457.

Hastings H, Cohen MS. General deep approaches: lateral approaches. Tech Shoulder Elbow Surg 2002;3:10–15.

NOTES

DISTAL BICEPS TENDON REPAIR, ENDOBUTTON

CPT code   24342 distal biceps tendon repair (endobutton)

ICD-9 code   727.62 rupture of biceps tendon, distal

INDICATIONS

- partial or complete distal biceps rupture
- prevent or treat painful or weak elbow flexion and supination in younger active patients

ALTERNATIVE TREATMENTS

- nonoperative treatment (older, less active patients)
- two-incision technique
- single incision, suture anchor
- single incision, interference screw

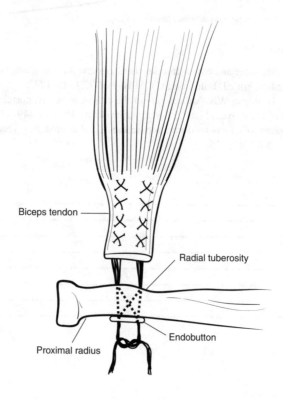

SURGICAL ANATOMY

Incision
- anterior transverse incision distal to elbow flexion crease

APPROACHES

Surgical Techniques
- identify and protect lateral antebrachial cutaneous nerve
- identify and tag biceps tendon stump proximally
- blunt dissection just medial to extensor wad (usually a tract left by avulsed tendon)
- protect recurrent leash of vessels as radial tuberosity exposed
- drill volar cortex to diameter of distal tendon
- drill posterior cortex with 4-mm endobutton drill
- weave two no. 5 sutures through tendon stump and secure endobutton 3–4 mm from end of stump
- pass endobutton–tendon complex with blunt needle
- flip and lock endobutton on dorsal cortex
- check position with mini-C arm

POSTOPERATIVE MANAGEMENT/REHABILITATION

- splint for 10 days, then begin passive flexion and active-assisted extension
- sling for 6 weeks
- begin supination and flexion strengthening at 12 weeks

COMPLICATIONS

- infection
- wound hematoma
- lateral antebrachial cutaneous nerve injury
- radial nerve injury (posterior interosseous nerve)
- radioulnar synostosis

SELECTED REFERENCES

Bain GI, Prem H, Hepinstall RJ, et al. Repair of distal biceps tendon rupture: a new technique using the Endobutton. J Shoulder Elbow Surg 2000;9:120–126.

Kelly EW, Morrey BF, O'Driscoll SW. Complications of repair of the distal biceps tendon with the modified two-incision technique. J Bone Joint Surg 2000;82A:1575–1581.

Galatz LM, Jani MM, Yamaguchi K. Single anterior incision exposure for distal biceps tendon repair. Tech Shoulder Elbow Surg 2002;3:63–67.

DISTAL BICEPS TENDON REPAIR, TWO-INCISION

CPT code   24342 distal biceps tendon repair (2-incision with trough)

ICD-9 code   727.62 rupture of biceps tendon, distal

INDICATIONS

- partial or complete distal biceps rupture
- prevent or treat painful or weak elbow flexion and supination in younger active patients

ALTERNATIVE TREATMENTS

- nonoperative treatment (older, less active patients)
- single incision, suture anchor
- single incision, endobutton
- single incision, interference screw

SURGICAL ANATOMY

Incision
- anterior, transverse skin incision distal to elbow flexion crease

APPROACHES

Surgical Techniques
- locate and protect lateral antebrachial cutaneous nerve
- find and tag distal biceps tendon with no. 5 suture
- blunt dissection to radial tuberosity following tract left by avulsed distal biceps tendon
- use hemostat to pass no. 5 suture just medial to radial tuberosity splitting extensor muscle dorsally
- make second skin incision dorsally over tip of hemostat
- bluntly split extensor muscles with forearm maximally pronated, deliver biceps tendon
- pronate forearm, expose radial tuberosity
- use burr and make a trough with drill holes
- secure tendon to bony trough

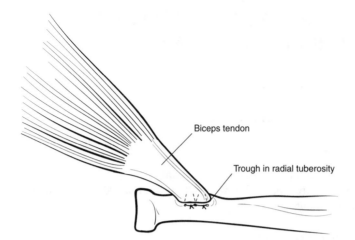

Biceps tendon

Trough in radial tuberosity

POSTOPERATIVE MANAGEMENT/REHABILITATION

- splint for 10 days then begin passive flexion, active-assisted extension
- sling for 6 weeks
- begin supination and flexion strengthening at 12 weeks

COMPLICATIONS

- infection
- wound hematoma
- lateral antebrachial cutaneous nerve injury
- radial nerve (posterior interosseous nerve) injury
- radioulnar synostosis

SELECTED REFERENCES

Kelly EW, Morrey BF, O'Driscoll SW. Complications of repair of the distal biceps tendon with the modified two-incision technique. J Bone Joint Surg Am 2000:82A:1575–1581.

Kelly EW, O'Driscoll SW. Mini-incision technique for acute distal biceps tendon repair. Tech Shoulder Elbow Surg 2002;3:57–62.

Morrey BF, Askew LJ, An KN, et al. Rupture of the distal tendon of the biceps brachii. A biomechanical study. J Bone Joint Surg Am 1985;67A:418–21.

DISTAL BICEPS TENDON REPAIR, SUTURE ANCHOR TECHNIQUE

CPT code   24342 distal biceps tendon repair (suture anchor technique)

ICD-9 code   727.62 rupture of biceps tendon, distal

INDICATIONS

- partial or complete distal biceps rupture
- prevent or treat painful or weak elbow flexion and supination in younger active patients

ALTERNATIVE TREATMENTS

- nonoperative treatment (older, less active patients)
- two-incision technique
- single incision, endobutton
- single incision, interference screw

SURGICAL ANATOMY

Incision
- anterior transverse incision distal to elbow flexion crease

APPROACHES

Surgical Techniques
- identify and protect lateral antebrachial cutaneous nerve
- identify and tag biceps tendon stump proximally
- blunt dissection just medial to extensor wad (usually a tract left by avulsed tendon)
- protect recurrent leash of vessels as radial tuberosity exposed
- place two suture anchors into radial tuberosity
- pass sutures from suture anchors into tendon and tie securely to bone

POSTOPERATIVE MANAGEMENT/REHABILITATION

- splint for 10 days then begin passive flexion and active-assisted extension
- sling for 6 weeks
- begin supination and flexion strengthening at 12 weeks

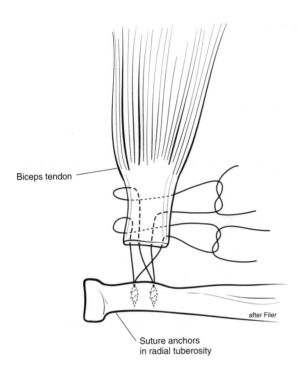

Biceps tendon

after Filer

Suture anchors
in radial tuberosity

COMPLICATIONS

- infection
- wound hematoma
- lateral antebrachial cutaneous nerve injury
- radial nerve injury (posterior interosseous nerve)
- radioulnar synostosis

SELECTED REFERENCES

Kelly EW, Morrey BF, O'Driscoll SW. Complications of repair of the distal biceps
    tendon with the modified two-incision technique. J Bone Joint Surg Am
    2000;82A:1575–1581.
Sotereanos DG, Pierce TD, Varitimidis SE. A simplified method for repair of distal
    biceps tendon ruptures. J Shoulder Elbow Surg 2000;9:227–233.
Galatz LM, Jani MM, Yamaguchi K. Single anterior incision exposure for distal
    biceps tendon repair. Tech Shoulder Elbow Surg 2002;3:63–67.

TRICEPS REPAIR

CPT code   24342 triceps repair

ICD-9 code   727.60 triceps tendon rupture

INDICATIONS

- complete or nearly complete avulsions or ruptures of triceps tendon

ALTERNATIVE TREATMENT

- nonoperative treatment in debilitated patients

SURGICAL ANATOMY

- prone position with injured arm resting on chest

Incision
- straight posterior, 10 cm above tip of olecranon to 3 cm below

APPROACHES

Surgical Techniques
- incise fascia
- drill 3-mm hole transversely through olecranon, 1 cm distal to tip
- pass two no. 5 Krackow-Thomas sutures (or 4-mm Mersilene tape) through tendon
- pass sutures through olecranon drill hole and tie with elbow in 30° of flexion

POSTOPERATIVE MANAGEMENT/REHABILITATION

- active-assisted ROM on first postoperative day
- splint for first 10 days
- full ROM attained by 6 weeks
- strengthening program at 8–10 weeks

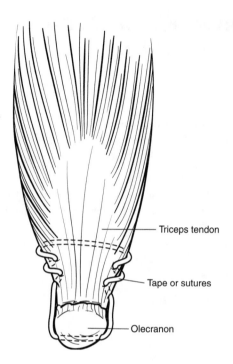

Triceps tendon

Tape or sutures

Olecranon

COMPLICATION

- wound infection

SELECTED REFERENCE

Levy M. Repair of triceps tendon avulsions or ruptures. J Bone Joint Surg Br 1987;69:115.

NOTES

RECONSTRUCTION OF LATERAL COLLATERAL LIGAMENT

CPT code   24344 reconstruction of lateral collateral ligament

ICD-9 codes   717.81 lateral collateral ligament
                      718.80 instability of elbow

INDICATIONS

- complete tear of the lateral ulnar collateral ligament (UCL) with resultant pain and instability of the elbow by characteristic lateral pivot shift clinically or under anesthesia
- positive imaging study, stress radiograph, or stress arthroscopy

ALTERNATIVE TREATMENT

- rest, NSAIDs, and rehabilitation

SURGICAL ANATOMY

Incision
- supine on arm board, tourniquet
- lateral skin incision, modified Kocher

APPROACH

- interval between triceps-anconeus and extensor mass

SURGICAL TECHNIQUES

- elevate common extensors and expose lateral UCL
- perform pivot shift and inspect quality of ligament
- expose supinator crest, create two tunnels with 7-mm bone bridge on ulna
- create humeral tunnel proximally on lateral epicondyle that exits near origin of ligament
- harvest palmaris longus tendon and pass
- secure by tying sutures and tendon strands together at 30° of elbow flexion with forearm pronated

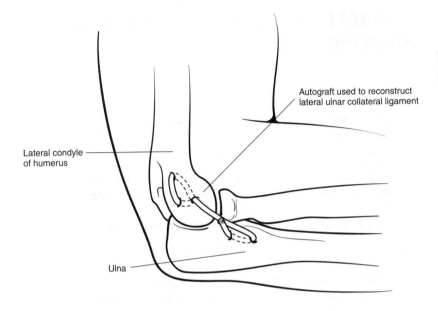

Autograft used to reconstruct
lateral ulnar collateral ligament

Lateral condyle
of humerus

Ulna

POSTOPERATIVE MANAGEMENT/REHABILITATION

- long-arm cast for 4 weeks, elbow at 90° of flexion with forearm in pronation
- hinged splint preventing extension past 30° for 6 weeks
- obtain full ROM and allow full activity after 4–6 months

COMPLICATIONS

- infection
- wound hematoma
- radial nerve injury
- recurrence of instability

SELECTED REFERENCES

Morrey BF, An KN. Articular and ligamentous contributions to the stability of the elbow joint. Am J Sports Med 1983;11:315–319.
Nestor BJ, O'Driscoll SW, Morrey BF. Ligamentous reconstruction for posterolateral rotatory instability of the elbow. J Bone Joint Surg Am 1992;74A:1235–1241.

REPAIR OF MEDIAL ULNAR COLLATERAL LIGAMENT

CPT code	**24345** repair of medial ulnar collateral ligament
ICD-9 code	**841.1** torn medial (ulnar) collateral ligament

INDICATIONS

- complete, acute avulsion of the UCL with excellent tissue quality
- partial tear of the UCL, unresponsive to nonoperative treatment in throwing athletes
- positive imaging study, stress radiograph, or stress arthroscopy

ALTERNATIVE TREATMENTS

- rest, NSAIDs, rehabilitation, throwing mechanics
- perform reconstruction with autograft using Jobe procedure, docking procedure, or interference screw

SURGICAL ANATOMY

- supine on arm board, tourniquet

Incision

- curvilinear incision over medial epicondyle

APPROACHES

Surgical Techniques

- protect medial antebrachial cutaneous nerve
- muscle-splitting incision of flexor mass
- elevate fibers from UCL and inspect ligament
- place "0" or no. 1 suture in Bunnell fashion and reattach through drill holes or use suture anchors
- if possible may be able to repair end-to-end or imbricate depending on injury pattern

POSTOPERATIVE MANAGEMENT/REHABILITATION

- posterior splint at 90° for 10–21 days
- active ROM after splint removed, begin strengthening at 6 weeks, avoid valgus stress for 4 months
- begin throwing program at 4 months

ELBOW

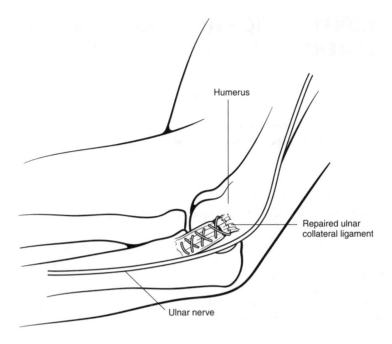

Humerus

Repaired ulnar collateral ligament

Ulnar nerve

COMPLICATIONS

- infection
- wound hematoma
- ulnar nerve injury
- recurrence of instability

SELECTED REFERENCES

Jobe FW, Stark H, Lombardo SJ. Reconstruction of the ulnar collateral ligament in athletes. J Bone Joint Surg Am 1986;68:1158–1163.

Morrey BF, An KN. Articular and ligamentous contributions to the stability of the elbow joint. Am J Sports Med 1983;11:315–319.

Conway JE, Jobe FW, Glousman RE, Pink M. Medial Instability of the elbow in throwing athletes. Treatment by repair or reconstruction of the ulnar collateral ligament. J Bone Joint Surg Am 1992;74A:67–83.

NOTES

RECONSTRUCTION OF MEDIAL COLLATERAL LIGAMENT, DOCKING PROCEDURE

CPT code	24346 reconstruction of medial collateral ligament, docking procedure

ICD-9 codes	718.1 instability of elbow
	841.1 medial (ulnar) collateral ligament

INDICATIONS

- complete tear of the UCL or
- partial tear of the UCL unresponsive to nonoperative treatment in throwing athletes
- positive imaging study, stress radiograph, or stress arthroscopy

ALTERNATIVE TREATMENTS

- rest, NSAIDs, rehabilitation, throwing mechanics
- Jobe procedure, 3-ply technique
- anatomic interference screw technique

SURGICAL ANATOMY

- supine on arm board, tourniquet

Incision
- curvilinear incision over medial epicondyle
- protect medial antebrachial cutaneous nerve
- muscle-splitting incision of flexor mass

APPROACHES

Surgical Techniques
- elevate fibers from UCL and then split ligament from epicondyle to sublime tubercle
- converging 3.2-mm drill holes create a tunnel in sublime tubercle leaving bone bridge
- drill single hole from distal to proximal with apex at ligament's origin on medial epicondyle
- drill two small holes into proximal aspect of humeral tunnel leaving a bone bridge
- harvest and pass palmaris longus tendon (fourth toe extensor or gracilis)
- tension the two free ends of the graft proximally and tie sutures over bone bridge with elbow at 60°

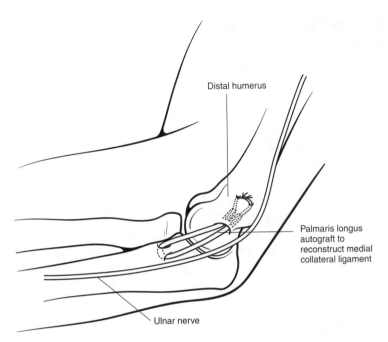

Distal humerus

Palmaris longus
autograft to
reconstruct medial
collateral ligament

Ulnar nerve

POSTOPERATIVE MANAGEMENT/REHABILITATION

- posterior splint at 90° for 10–21 days
- active ROM after splint removed, begin strengthening at 6 weeks, avoid valgus stress for 4 months
- begin throwing program at 4 months

COMPLICATIONS

- infection
- wound hematoma
- ulnar nerve injury
- recurrence of instability

SELECTED REFERENCES

Morrey BF, An KN. Articular and ligamentous contributions to the stability of the elbow joint. Am J Sports Med 1983;11:315–319.

Elattrache N, Bast SC, David T. Medial collateral ligament reconstruction. Tech Shoulder Elbow Surg 2001;2:38–49.

RECONSTRUCTION OF MEDIAL COLLATERAL LIGAMENT, ANATOMIC INTERFERENCE SCREW

CPT code	24346 reconstruction of medial collateral ligament, anatomic IF screw

ICD-9 codes	718.80 instability of elbow
	841.1 instability of elbow

INDICATIONS

- complete tear or partial tear of UCL
- treatment in throwing athletes
- positive imaging study, stress radiograph or stress arthroscopy

ALTERNATIVE TREATMENTS

- rest, NSAIDs, and rehabilitation
- throwing mechanics
- Jobe procedure, 3-ply technique
- "docking procedure"

SURGICAL ANATOMY

- supine on arm board, tourniquet

Incision

- curvilinear incision over medial epicondyle

APPROACHES

Surgical Techniques

- protect medial antebrachial cutaneous nerve
- muscle-splitting incision of flexor mass
- elevate fibers from UCL and then split ligament from epicondyle to sublime tubercle
- drill 4-mm diameter hole in sublime tubercle over guide pin, angled 45°, 5 mm from articular surface
- drill guide pin into medial epicondyle retrograde—should exit epicondyle anterior to intermuscular septum, drill 4-mm tunnel
- harvest and pass palmaris longus tendon
- fold tendon into 3-ply construct
- seat graft fully into ulnar tunnel, place 5-mm screw
- pass graft proximally, tension at 60°, and secure with 5-mm screw

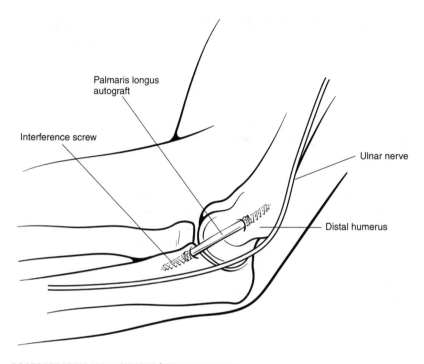

Palmaris longus
autograft

Interference screw

Ulnar nerve

Distal humerus

POSTOPERATIVE MANAGEMENT/REHABILITATION

- hand-grip exercises, immobilize for 10–21 days
- active ROM after splint removed, begin strengthening at 6 weeks, avoid valgus stress for 4 months
- begin throwing program at 4 months

COMPLICATIONS

- infection
- wound hematoma
- ulnar nerve injury
- recurrence of instability

SELECTED REFERENCES

Jobe FW, Stark H, Lombardo SJ. Reconstruction of the ulnar collateral ligament in athletes. J Bone Joint Surg 1986;68:1158–1163.
Elattrache N, Bast SC, David T. Medial collateral ligament reconstruction. Tech Shoulder Elbow Surg 2001;2:38–49.

RECONSTRUCTION OF MEDIAL COLLATERAL LIGAMENT, 3-PLY OR JOBE PROCEDURE

CPT code 24346 reconstruction of medial collateral ligament, 3-ply or Jobe procedure

ICD-9 codes 718.80 instability of elbow
841.1 medial (ulnar) collateral ligament

INDICATIONS

- complete tear of the ulnar collateral ligament (UCL)
- partial tear of the UCL unresponsive to nonoperative treatment in throwing athletes
- positive imaging study, stress radiograph, or stress arthroscopy

ALTERNATIVE TREATMENTS

- rest, NSAIDs, rehabilitation, throwing mechanics
- docking procedure
- anatomic interference (IF) screw technique

SURGICAL ANATOMY

- supine on arm board, tourniquet

Incision
- curvilinear incision over medial epicondyle

APPROACHES

Surgical Techniques
- protect medial antebrachial cutaneous nerve
- muscle-splitting incision of flexor mass
- elevate fibers from UCL and then split ligament from epicondyle to sublime tubercle
- converging 3.2-mm drill holes create a tunnel in sublime tubercle leaving bone bridge
- divergent drill holes from distal to proximal with apex at ligament's origin on medial epicondyle
- harvest and pass palmaris longus tendon (or fourth toe extensor, gracilis)
- tension at 60° and suture limbs near mouths of each tunnel incorporating native UCL

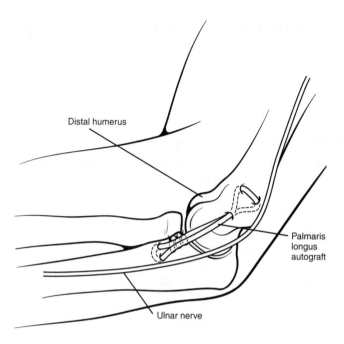

Distal humerus

Palmaris
longus
autograft

Ulnar nerve

POSTOPERATIVE MANAGEMENT/REHABILITATION

- posterior splint at 90° for 10–21 days
- active ROM after splint removed, begin strengthening at 6 weeks, avoid valgus stress for 4 months
- begin throwing program at 4 months

COMPLICATIONS

- infection
- wound hematoma
- ulnar nerve injury
- recurrence of instability

SELECTED REFERENCES

Jobe FW, Stark H, Lombardo SJ. Reconstruction of the ulnar collateral ligament in athletes. J Bone Joint Surg 1986;68:1158–1163.

Morrey BF, An KN. Articular and ligamentous contributions to the stability of the elbow joint. Am J Sports Med 1983;11:315–319.

Elattrache NS, Bast SC, David T. Medial collateral ligament reconstruction. Tech Shoulder Elbow Surg 2001;2:38–49.

DEBRIDEMENT OF LATERAL EPICONDYLE

CPT code   24350 debridement of lateral epicondyle

ICD-9 code   726.32 lateral epicondylitis

INDICATIONS

Chronic lateral elbow pain over lateral epicondyle despite rehabilitation, NSAIDs, corticosteroid injections, and bracing.

ALTERNATIVE TREATMENTS

- release of extensor radialis brevis
- arthroscopic debridement

SURGICAL ANATOMY

Incision
- lateral skin incision over epicondyle

APPROACHES

Surgical Techniques
- incise extensor fascia between extensor digitorum communis (EDC) and ECRL
- split extensor carpi radialis brevis (ECRB) and look for yellow-gray mucoid degenerative tissue
- excise degenerative tissue and drill epicondyle with small drill to promote bleeding bed

REHABILITATION

- sling for 7–10 days
- gentle, active-assisted ROM
- extensor strengthening

COMPLICATIONS

- infection
- wound hematoma
- nerve injury (with lateral approach)

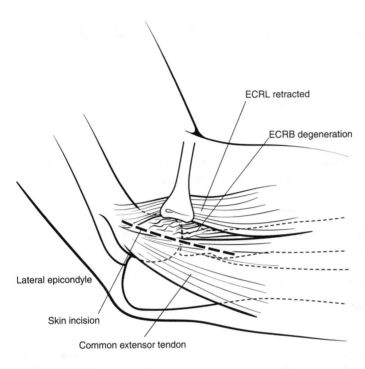

ECRL retracted

ECRB degeneration

Lateral epicondyle

Skin incision

Common extensor tendon

SELECTED REFERENCE

Nirschl RP, Pettrone FA. Tennis elbow. The surgical treatment of lateral epicondylitis. J Bone Joint Surg Am 1979;61A:832–839.

NOTES

RELEASE OF EXTENSOR TENDON ORIGIN

CPT code   24350 release of extensor tendon origin

ICD-9 code   726.32 lateral epicondylitis

INDICATIONS

Chronic lateral elbow pain over lateral epicondyle, despite rehabilitation, NSAIDs, corticosteroid injections, and bracing.

ALTERNATIVE TREATMENTS

* open debridement of extensor carpi radialis brevis (ECRB)
* arthroscopic debridement

APPROACHES

* prone position, elbow flexed to 90°

Surgical Techniques

* infiltrate skin and subcutaneous tissue with 1% Xylocaine/epinephrine
* no. 11 blade, 2-mm anterior to tip of epicondyle, keep blade parallel to long axis of humerus
* release ECRB
* ask patient to flex and extend wrist
* rasp epicondyle, apply soft dressing

POSTOPERATIVE MANAGEMENT/REHABILITATION

* sling for comfort for 3–7 days
* active-assisted ROM, active ROM, and PREs

COMPLICATIONS

* infection
* wound hematoma
* radial nerve injury (with lateral approach)

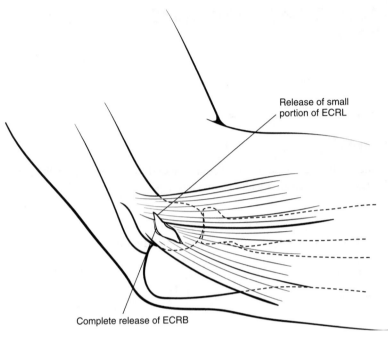

Release of small
portion of ECRL

Complete release of ECRB

SELECTED REFERENCE

Savoie FH. Percutaneous release for lateral epicondylitis. Tech Shoulder Elbow Surg
2001;2:243–246.

NOTES

FASCIECTOMY, DEBRIDEMENT OF MEDIAL EPICONDYLE

CPT code   24350 fasciectomy, debridement of medial epicondyle

ICD-9 code   726.31 medial epicondylitis

INDICATIONS

Chronic medial elbow pain over medial epicondyle, despite rehabilitation, NSAIDs, corticosteroid injections, and bracing.

ALTERNATIVE TREATMENTS

* rest, NSAIDs, bracing, common flexor rehabilitation

SURGICAL ANATOMY

* supine position

Incision

* medial skin incision over epicondyle and common flexors

APPROACHES

Surgical Techniques

* incise common flexor distal to epicondyle
* reflect common flexor but preserve medial collateral ligament, may split common flexor also
* excise degenerative tissue on undersurface of pronator and drill epicondyle with small drill to promote bleeding bed
* reattach common flexors

POSTOPERATIVE MANAGEMENT/REHABILITATION

* sling for 7–10 days
* gentle active-assisted ROM
* extensor strengthening at 4–6 weeks

COMPLICATIONS

* infection
* wound hematoma
* ulnar nerve injury
* disruption of the medial collateral ligament

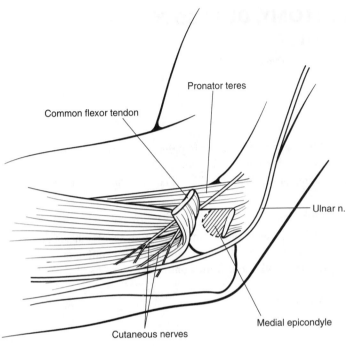

Pronator teres

Common flexor tendon

Ulnar n.

Medial epicondyle

Cutaneous nerves

SELECTED REFERENCES

Nirschl RP, Pettrone FA. Tennis elbow. The surgical treatment of lateral epicondylitis. J Bone Joint Surg Am 1979;61A:832–839.

Jobe FW, Ciccotti MG. Lateral and medial epicondylitis of the elbow. J Am Acad Orthop Surg 1994;2:1–8.

NOTES

ARTHROSCOPY OF ELBOW

CPT code   **28766 arthroscopy of elbow**

ICD-9 code   **718.12 loose body, elbow**

INDICATIONS

- mechanical locking, catching, and popping with elbow motion, not relieved with rest, rehabilitation, or NSAIDs
- positive imaging study: radiographs, CT arthrography, or MRI

OTHER INDICATIONS

- excision olecranon osteophytes, synovectomy, lysis of adhesions
- debridement, drilling osteochondritis dissecans of capitellum
- release of posttraumatic or arthritic contractures

ALTERNATIVE TREATMENT

- open arthrotomy

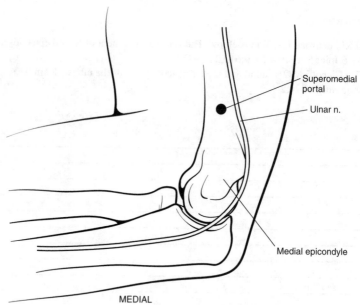

From Stubbs MJ, Field LD, Savoie FH: Osteochondritis dissecans of the elbow. Clin Sports Med 2001;20(1): 6, Figures C,D.

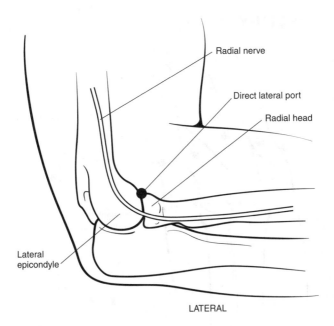

ELBOW

Radial nerve

Direct lateral port

Radial head

Lateral
epicondyle

LATERAL

SURGICAL ANATOMY/SET UP

- general anesthesia, tourniquet
- supine
- prone
- lateral decubitus

Portals

- proximal medial: 2 cm proximal to medial epicondyle, anterior to intermuscular septum
- anterolateral and direct lateral ("soft spot")
- posterolateral
- posterocentral

APPROACHES

Surgical Techniques

- 4.0 mm, 2.7 mm arthroscopes and shavers, hand instruments
- instill joint with 10 mL saline through "soft spot"
- scope into superomedial portal
- shaver, hand instruments through lateral portal
- switch scope to lateral portal and instruments to medial
- scope and instruments to posterior lateral and posterior central

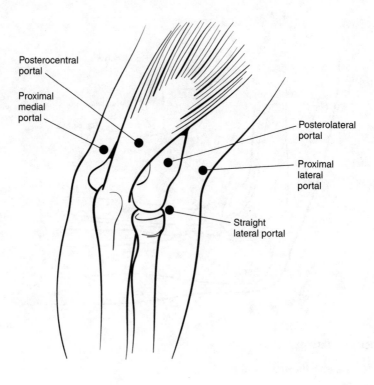

Posterocentral
portal

Proximal
medial
portal

Posterolateral
portal

Proximal
lateral
portal

Straight
lateral portal

POSTOPERATIVE MANAGEMENT/REHABILITATION

- sling for comfort for 1–3 days and then motion
- passive ROM, active ROM, and PREs

COMPLICATIONS

- infection
- wound hematoma
- radial nerve injury (with lateral portal), ulnar nerve injury

SELECTED REFERENCES

Baker CL, Jones GL. Arthroscopy of the elbow. Am J Sports Med 1999;27:251–264.
Stother K, Day B, Regan WR. Arthroscopy of the elbow: anatomy, portal sites, and a description of the proximal lateral portal. Arthroscopy 1995;11:449–457.

NOTES

_____

_____

_____

_____

_____

ARTHROSCOPY OF ELBOW, OSTEOARTICULAR TRANSFER TO CAPITELLUM

CPT code   29999 arthroscopy of elbow, loose body removal, debridement, osteoarticular
                         transfer to capitellum

ICD-9 code   732.3 Panner's disease
                  732.7 osteochondritis dissecans of capitellum

INDICATIONS

- mechanical locking, catching, and popping with elbow motion not relieved with rest, rehabilitation, and NSAIDs
- positive imaging study: radiographs, CT arthrography, or MRI

ALTERNATIVE TREATMENTS

- open arthrotomy to debride, curettage lesion
- arthroscopic microfracture chondroplasty
- humeral osteotomy

SURGICAL ANATOMY

- supine
- prone
- lateral decubitus

Portals

- anteromedial
- lateral
- posterolateral
- posterocentral

APPROACHES

Surgical Techniques

- instill joint with 10 mL saline through "soft spot"
- scope into superomedial portal
- shaver, hand instruments through lateral portal
- debride lesion, measure and prepare site for osteoarticular transfer
- arthroscopy of knee to harvest donor osteoarticular plug (alternative donor, allograft)
- resurface capitellum arthroscopically or by lateral arthrotomy

ELBOW

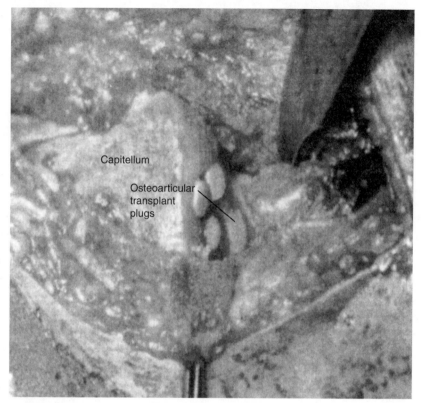

Capitellum

Osteoarticular
transplant
plugs

From Nakagawa et al.

POSTOPERATIVE MANAGEMENT/REHABILITATION

- sling for comfort for 1–3 days and then motion
- passive ROM, active ROM, no resistance strengthening for 4–6 weeks

COMPLICATIONS

- infection
- wound hematoma
- radial nerve injury (with lateral approach)

SELECTED REFERENCES

Ruch DS, Poehling GG. Arthroscopic treatment of Panner's disease. Clin Sports Med 1991;10:629–636.
Schenck RC Jr, Goodnight JM. Osteochondritis dissecans [Current Concepts Review] J Bone Joint Surg Am 1996;78A:439–456.
Nakagawa Y, Matsusue Y, Ikeda N, et al. Osteochondral grafting and arthroplasty for end-stage osteochondritis dissecans of the capitellum. Am J Sports Med 2001;29: 650–655.

ARTHROSCOPY OF ELBOW, LATERAL DISTAL HUMERAL OSTEOTOMY

CPT code   24400 and 29999 arthroscopy of elbow, loose body removal, debridement, lateral distal humeral osteotomy

ICD-9 code   723.3 Panner's disease

              732.7 osteochondritis dissecans of capitellum

INDICATIONS

- mechanical locking, catching, and popping with elbow motion not relieved with rest, rehabilitation, or NSAIDs
- positive imaging study: radiographs, CT-arthrography, or MRI

ALTERNATIVE TREATMENTS

- open arthrotomy to debride, curettage lesion
- arthroscopic microfracture chondroplasty
- osteoarticular transfer to capitellum (auto-allograft)

SURGICAL ANATOMY

- supine
- prone
- lateral decubitus

Portals

- anteromedial
- lateral
- posterolateral
- posterocentral

APPROACHES

Surgical Techniques

- instill joint with 10 mL saline through "soft spot"
- scope into superomedial portal
- shaver, hand instruments through lateral portal
- debride lesion, inspect posteriorly for loose bodies
- lateral approach to distal humerus, Kocher approach
- osteotomize distal humerus, lateral column from proximal-lateral to distal-medial, creating 10° closing wedge
- stabilize with internal fixation

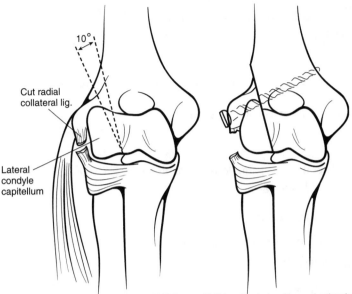

10°

Cut radial
collateral lig.

Lateral
condyle
capitellum

From Nakagawa Y, Matsusue Y, Ikeda N, Asada Y, Nakamura T: Osteochondral grafting and arthroplasty for
end-stage osteochrondritis dissecans of the capitellum. Am J Sports Med 2001;29(5):p.652, Figure 3C.

POSTOPERATIVE MANAGEMENT/REHABILITATION

- splint for comfort for 5–7 days and then motion
- passive ROM, active-assisted ROM
- no resistance strengthening for 4–6 weeks
- restrict activity until radiographic union of osteotomy site

COMPLICATIONS

- infection
- wound hematoma
- radial nerve injury (with lateral approach)

SELECTED REFERENCES

Ruch DS, Poehling GG. Arthroscopic treatment of Panner's disease. Clin Sports Med
    1991;10:629–636.
Schenck RC Jr, Goodnight JM. Osteochondritis dissecans [Current Concepts Review]
    J Bone Joint Surg Am 1996;78A:439–456.
Kiyoshige Y, Takagi M, Yuasa K, et al. Closed-wedged osteotomy for osteochondritis
    dissecans of the capitellum. Am J Sports Med 2000;28:534–537.

ARTHROSCOPIC DEBRIDEMENT, RELEASE OF LATERAL EPICONDYLE

CPT code   29999 arthroscopic debridement/release of lateral epicondyle

ICD-9 code   726.32 lateral epicondylitis

INDICATIONS

Chronic lateral elbow pain, despite rehabilitation, NSAIDs, corticosteroid injections, and bracing.

ALTERNATIVE TREATMENTS

- release of extensor carpi radialis brevis
- open debridement

SURGICAL ANATOMY

- prone
- supine
- lateral decubitus

APPROACHES

Surgical Techniques
- distension of elbow with 20 mL saline
- make skin incision proximal medial portal, 2 cm proximal and 2 cm anterior to medial epicondyle
- use hemostat to bluntly spread subcutaneous tissue
- arthroscope medially
- establish proximal lateral portal and perform diagnostic arthroscopy
- push scope past radial head and observe ECRB in front of camera
- use 4.5-mm shaver from lateral and debride capsule and ECRB
- decorticate lateral epicondyle with 3–4-mm burr

POSTOPERATIVE MANAGEMENT/REHABILITATION

- sling for comfort 3–5 days
- active-assisted ROM, active ROM, and PREs

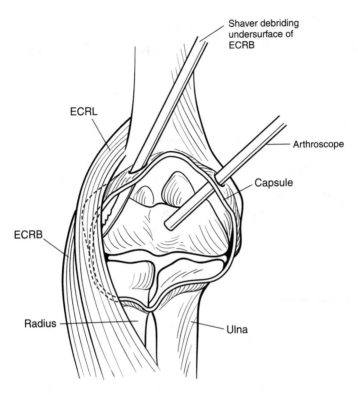

COMPLICATIONS

- infection
- wound hematoma
- radial nerve injury

SELECTED REFERENCES

Baker CL, Kuklo TR, Taylor KR, et al. Arthroscopic release for lateral epicondylitis: a cadaveric model. Arthroscopy 1999;15:259–264.
Owens BD, Murphy KP, Kuklo TR. Arthroscopic release for lateral epicondylitis. Arthroscopy 2001;17:582–587.

NOTES

ARTHROSCOPIC RESECTION, POSTERIOR MEDIAL OLECRANON IMPINGEMENT

CPT code	29999 arthroscopic resection, posterior medial olecranon impingement

ICD-9 codes	718.82 elbow derangement (posterior elbow impingement, valgus extension overload)

INDICATIONS

- pain, stiffness, locking, usually seen in throwing athletes
- failure of nonsurgical management

ALTERNATIVE TREATMENT

- open resection

SURGICAL ANATOMY

- patient prone with shoulder abducted to 90°, and arm supported by arm positioner, allowing elbow to rest in 90° of flexion

Portals

- straight lateral, posterocentral, proximal anterolateral, proximal anteromedial

APPROACHES

Surgical Techniques

- excision of trochlear spurs and debridement
- proximal anteromedial portal used for synovectomy, radiocapitellar joint debridement, coronoid osteophyte excision, and deepening of coronoid fossa
- evaluation of posterior compartment with posterolateral and posterocentral portals
- evaluation of medial and lateral gutters—excise adhesions, debridement
- debridement of olecranon fossa if narrowed (by bony hypertrophy, loose bodies, and scar tissue)
- drains in proximal anteromedial and the posterocentral or posterolateral portals
- closure of straight lateral portal
- other portals left open

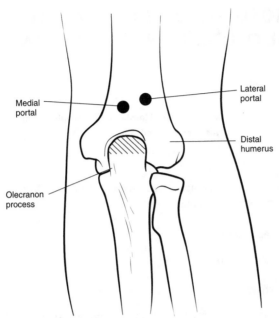

POSTOPERATIVE MANAGEMENT/REHABILITATION

- early motion with or without continuous passive motion (CPM)
- static splinting of CPM for at least 3 weeks postoperatively, if motion gain is significant goal
- throwers: begin strengthening with low-weight, high-repetition isotonic exercises

COMPLICATIONS

- nerve injury (ulnar)
- recurrence in high-demand overhand athletes

SELECTED REFERENCES

Cain EL, Andrews JR. Arthroscopic management of posterior elbow impingement in throwers. Tech Shoulder Elbow Surg 2001;2:118–130.
Lyons TR, Field LD, Savoie FH. Instr Course Lect 2000;49:239–246.

NOTES

_____
_____
_____
_____
_____

ARTHROTOMY, RESECTION, POSTERIOR MEDIAL OLECRANON IMPINGEMENT

CPT code   29999 arthrotomy, resection, posterior medial olecranon impingement

ICD-9 code   718.82 elbow derangement (posterior elbow impingement,
                        valgus extension overload)

INDICATIONS

- pain, stiffness, and locking, usually seen in throwing athletes
- failure of nonsurgical management

ALTERNATIVE TREATMENT

- arthroscopic resection

SURGICAL ANATOMY

- prone position, shoulder abducted to 90°, and arm supported by arm positioner, allowing elbow to rest in 90° of flexion

Incision

- posterolateral incision, develop interval between anconeus and extensor carpi ulnaris

APPROACHES

Surgical Techniques

- excision of trochlear spurs and debridement
- debridement of olecranon fossa, if narrowed (by bony hypertrophy, loose bodies, and scar tissue)
- osteotome to resect osteophyte

POSTOPERATIVE MANAGEMENT/REHABILITATION

- splint in extension and supination
- early motion with or without continuous passive motion (CPM)
- static splinting of CPM for at least 3 weeks postoperatively if motion gain is significant goal
- throwers: begin strengthening with low-weight, high-repetition isotonic exercises

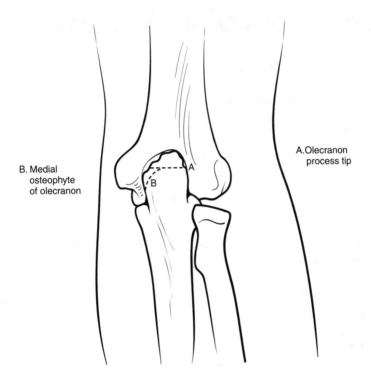

B. Medial
osteophyte
of olecranon

A.Olecranon
process tip

COMPLICATIONS

- nerve injury (ulnar)
- recurrence in high-demand overhand athletes

SELECTED REFERENCE

Wilson FD, Andrews JR, Blackburn TA, et al. Valgus extension overload in the
pitching elbow. Am J Sports Med 1983;11:83–88.

NOTES

_____

_____

_____

_____

ARTHROSCOPIC CAPSULAR RELEASE

CPT code   29999 arthroscopic capsular release

ICD-9 code   718.42 elbow contracture

INDICATIONS

- loss of elbow extension of greater than 30°
- extension loss secondary to intra-articular causes, such as posttraumatic
- failed rehabilitation, dynamic splinting

CONTRAINDICATIONS

- altered neurovascular anatomy, previous ulnar nerve transposition, or subluxing ulnar nerve

ALTERNATIVE TREATMENTS

- lateral column procedure
- external fixator lengthening
- arthrotomy, capsulectomy/release

SURGICAL ANATOMY

- prone
- supine
- lateral decubitus

APPROACHES

Surgical Techniques
- mark skin for bony anatomy, use tourniquet
- use soft spot and insufflate with saline
- proximal medial portal with scope, debride from lateral portal, release anterior capsule laterally
- switch portals and release medial capsule
- create posterocentral and posterolateral portals
- debride posterior joint, resect posterior olecranon osteophytes
- in severe cases consider ulnohumeral arthroplasty enlarging olecranon fossa

POSTOPERATIVE MANAGEMENT/REHABILITATION

- CPM, extension orthosis

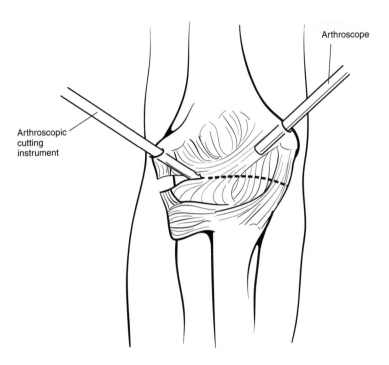

COMPLICATIONS

- infection
- wound hematoma
- radial, ulnar, and median nerve injury

SELECTED REFERENCES

Husband JB, Hastings HH. The lateral approach for operative release of post-traumatic contracture of the elbow. J Bone Joint Surg 1990;72:1353–1358.
Noojin FK, Savoie FH, Field LD. Arthroscopic release of the stiff elbow. Tech Shoulder Elbow Surg 2001;2:17–26.

NOTES

KNEE

ARTHROTOMY, WITH EXPLORATION, DRAINAGE, OR FOREIGN BODY REMOVAL

CPT code	27310 arthrotomy, knee, with exploration, drainage, or removal of foreign body (e.g., infection)
ICD-9 code	711.06 septic
	717.6 loose body arthritis
	718.36 internal derangement

INDICATIONS

- deep infection involving knee joint
- loose body, foreign body

ALTERNATIVE TREATMENTS

- arthroscopic incision and drainage
- serial aspirations in debilitated patients or others not able to undergo surgical procedures
- intravenous antibiotics (usually utilized in addition to the aforementioned treatments)

SURGICAL ANATOMY

Incision
- incision is midline, which allows for future procedures
- anteromedial or lateral capsulotomy
- secondary incisions to remove or debride abscesses also should be made to allow complete removal of infection

APPROACH

- supine, except for isolated posterior fossa abscesses

SURGICAL TECHNIQUE

- debride all infected tissue to reduce overall bacterial count to as low as possible

POSTOPERATIVE MANAGEMENT

- intravenous antibiotics followed by oral coverage for total of 6 weeks, depending on virulence of bacteria and completeness of debridement

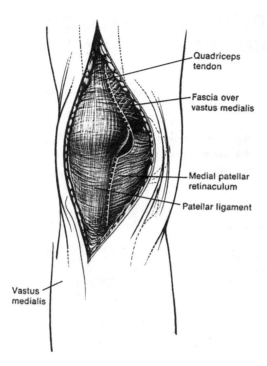

Quadriceps tendon

Fascia over vastus medialis

Medial patellar retinaculum

Patellar ligament

Vastus medialis

REHABILITATION

- begin range of motion (ROM) and strengthening after incision has healed
- initially quadriceps activation and patellar mobilization should be undertaken

COMPLICATIONS

- inadequate debridement allowing ongoing infection
- synovial fistula

SELECTED REFERENCES

Lane JG, Falahee MH, Wojtys EM, Hankin FM, Kaufer H. Pyarthrosis of the knee. Clin Orthop 1990;252:198–204.
Wirtz DC, Marth M, Miltner O, Schneider U, Zilkens KW. Septic arthritis of the knee in adults: treatment by arthroscopy or arthrotomy. Int Orthop 2001;25:239–241.

ARTHROTOMY, WITH EXCISION OF SEMILUNAR CARTILAGE (MENISCECTOMY)

CPT code   27332 arthrotomy, with excision of semilunar cartilage (meniscectomy) knee; medial OR lateral

ICD-9 codes   718.36 internal derangement
836.0 medial meniscus tear
836.1 lateral meniscus tear

INDICATIONS

- torn medial or lateral meniscus

ALTERNATIVE TREATMENTS

- arthroscopic meniscectomy (CPT code 29881)
- observation
- activity modification

SURGICAL ANATOMY

- oblique arthrotomy at joint line

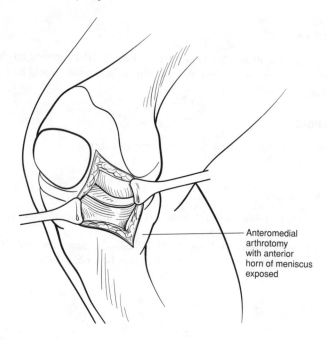

Anteromedial arthrotomy with anterior horn of meniscus exposed

INCISIONS

- midline skin incision to medial retinaculum with parapatellar arthrotomy
- incision to capsule and then through to meniscal-capsular junction

APPROACHES

Surgical Techniques

- incise anterior horn from capsule and grasp
- continue incision of meniscocapsular junction posteriorly using curved blades or meniscotomes
- for retained posterior horn may have to make posterior arthrotomy
- second incision posterior to posterior border of medial collateral ligament, incise pes fascia and protect saphenous nerve
- expose posteromedial capsule and make vertical arthrotomy to expose posterior horn
- excise posterior horn

KNEE

POSTOPERATIVE MANAGEMENT

- crutches for safety
- pain medication as required
- deep vein thrombosis (DVT) prophylaxis when indicated

REHABILITATION

- ROM immediately to prevent stiffness
- strengthening once ROM re-established
- wean from crutches when gait normalized

COMPLICATIONS

- postoperative infection
- progression of arthritic changes
- exacerbation of arthritic condition (10%)

SELECTED REFERENCES

Hoppenfeld S, DeBoer P. In: Surgical exposures in orthopaedics: the anatomic approach. Philadelphia: JB Lippincott, 1984:396–400.
Hamberg P, Gillquist J, Lysholm J. A comparison between arthroscopic meniscectomy and modified open meniscectomy. A prospective randomized study. J Bone Joint Surg Br 1984;66:189–192.

ARTHROTOMY, WITH SYNOVECTOMY, ANTERIOR OR POSTERIOR

CPT code	27334 arthrotomy, with synovectomy, knee; anterior OR posterior

ICD-9 codes	286.0 hemophilia
	714.0 rheumatoid arthritis
	719.26 pigmented villonodular synovitis
	727.82 synovial osteochondromatosis

INDICATIONS

- rheumatoid arthritis with significant synovial involvement, unable to be treated by conservative methods including injections
- generalized synovitis secondary to inflammatory arthritic disease, unable to be treated by conservative methods including injections

ALTERNATIVE TREATMENTS

- conservative care to include NSAIDs, oral steroids, corticosteroid injections
- activity modification
- radiosynovectomy with use of P-32 or other radioactive substances
- arthroscopic synovectomy

SURGICAL ANATOMY

Incision
- utility incision is midline

APPROACHES

Surgical Techniques
- incise medial retinaculum and capsule, extend proximally and split quadriceps tendon to permit dislocation of patella, debride synovium
- direct posterior incision via lazy-"S" incision for isolated posterior synovectomy (patient prone)
- divide deep fascia and develop interval between medial and lateral heads of gastrocnemius, isolate and protect tibial nerve and popliteal artery and vein
- arthrotomy with sharp debridement or curettage (or both) of involved synovial lining

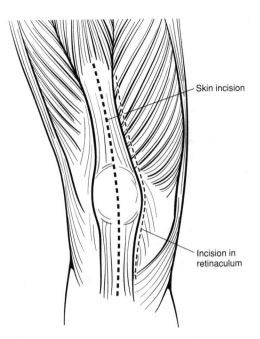

Skin incision

Incision in
retinaculum

KNEE

POSTOPERATIVE MANAGEMENT

- crutches for safety
- pain medication as needed
- prophylactic or additional NSAIDs or steroid treatment (or both) as adjunct for severe cases

REHABILITATION

- ROM and strengthening as possible
- consider aqua therapy for extensive debridements

COMPLICATIONS

- recurrent inflammatory disease in severe cases or after incomplete resection

SELECTED REFERENCES

Hoppenfeld S, DeBoer P. Surgical exposures in orthopaedics: the anatomic approach. Philadelphia: JB Lippincott, 1984:390–394.

Ishikawa H, Ohno O, Hirohata K. Long-term results of synovectomy in rheumatoid patients. J Bone Joint Surg Am 1986;68:198–205.

ARTHROTOMY, WITH SYNOVECTOMY, ANTERIOR AND POSTERIOR

CPT code	27335 arthrotomy, with synovectomy, knee; anterior AND posterior including popliteal area

ICD-9 codes	714.0 rheumatoid arthritis
	719.26 pigmented villonodular synovitis
	727.82 synovial osteochondromatosis

INDICATIONS

- rheumatoid arthritis with significant synovial involvement, unable to be treated by conservative methods including injections
- generalized synovitis secondary to inflammatory arthritic disease, unable to be treated by conservative methods including injections

ALTERNATIVE TREATMENTS

- conservative care to include NSAIDs, oral steroids, and corticosteroid injections
- activity modification
- radiosynovectomy with use of P-32 or other radioactive substances
- arthroscopic synovectomy

SURGICAL ANATOMY

Incision
- utility incision is midline

APPROACHES

Surgical Techniques
- direct posterior incision via lazy-"S" incision for cases requiring more-extensive posterior synovectomy
- arthrotomy with sharp debridement or curettage (or both) of involved synovial lining

POSTOPERATIVE MANAGEMENT

- crutches for safety
- pain medication as needed
- prophylactic or additional NSAID or steroid treatment (or both) as adjunct for severe cases

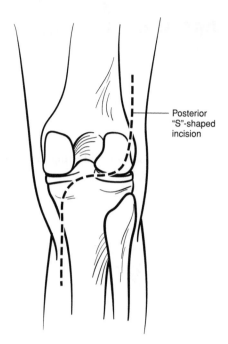

Posterior
"S"-shaped
incision

REHABILITATION

- ROM and strengthening as possible
- consider aqua therapy for extensive debridements

COMPLICATIONS

- continued inflammatory disease in severe cases or after incomplete resection

SELECTED REFERENCES

Hoppenfeld S, DeBoer P. Surgical exposures in orthopaedics: the anatomic approach. Philadelpha: JB Lippincott, 1984:390–394.
Triantafyllou SJ, Hanks GA, Handal JA, Greer RB 3rd. Open and arthroscopic synovectomy in hemophilic arthropathy of the knee. Clin Orthop 1992;283:196–204.

NOTES

EXCISION, PREPATELLAR BURSA

CPT code   27340 excision, prepatellar bursa

ICD-9 code   726.65 chronic prepatellar bursitis

INDICATIONS

- chronic or recalcitrant bursal swelling affecting function
- infected prepatellar bursa

ALTERNATIVE TREATMENTS

- observation
- aspiration, single or recurrent, with or without corticosteroid injection

SURGICAL ANATOMY

Incision
- midline over bursa
- alternate: transverse incision over patella

APPROACHES

Surgical Techniques
- develop plane: bursa, skin, and patella
- deep incision to patellar periosteum
- excision of entire bursa including cyst lining

POSTOPERATIVE MANAGEMENT

- temporary immobilization to prevent hematoma
- crutches as needed
- pain medication as needed
- antibiotics for severely infected bursa

REHABILITATION

- ROM and strengthening after ROM established

COMPLICATIONS

- incomplete resection causing recurrence
- postoperative infection
- synovial fistula

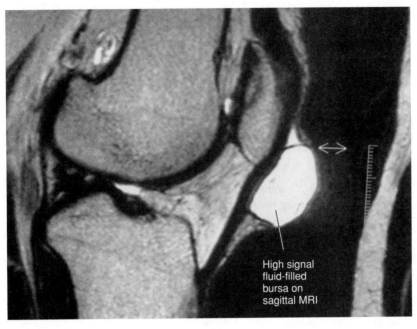

KNEE

High signal
fluid-filled
bursa on
sagittal MRI

SELECTED REFERENCES

Cox JS, Blanda JB. Peripatellar pathologies. In: DeLee JC, Drez D, Miller M, eds. Orthopaedic sports medicine, 1st ed. Philadelphia: WB Saunders, 1994:1249–1250.
Justis EJ. Nontraumatic disorders. In: Crenshaw AH, ed. Campbell's operative orthopaedics, 7th ed. St. Louis: CV Mosby, 1987:2252–2254.

NOTES

EXCISION OF SYNOVIAL CYST OF POPLITEAL SPACE

CPT code	**27345** excision of synovial cyst of popliteal space (e.g. Baker's cyst)
ICD-9 code	**727.41** ganglion
	727.51 synovial cyst (Baker's cyst)

INDICATIONS

- popliteal cyst, recalcitrant to conservative measures
- popliteal cyst, causing neurologic or vascular compromise to lower leg

ALTERNATIVE TREATMENTS

- observation
- activity modification
- aspiration and injection with corticosteroids, either cyst itself or intra-articular space (or both)
- arthroscopic resection

SURGICAL ANATOMY

Incision
- posterior lazy-"S" incision over cyst

APPROACHES

Surgical Techniques
- develop interval between medial head of gastrocnemius and semimembranosus to expose cyst
- dissection should be done following knee arthrotomy or arthroscopy to address intra-articular pathology because primary cause of cyst is sequelae of meniscal tear
- intra-articular or intra-cystic injection of methylene blue to better identify and locate cyst
- complete cyst excision, including cyst wall

POSTOPERATIVE MANAGEMENT

- pain medication and antibiotics as needed
- crutches for safety

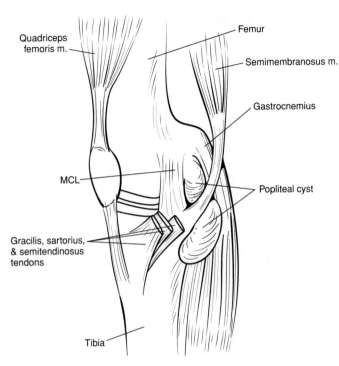

KNEE

REHABILITATION

- ROM and strengthening after motion established

COMPLICATIONS

- loss of knee motion
- postoperative infection
- recurrent cyst formation secondary to treat cyst etiology intra-articularly or to completely remove cyst wall

SELECTED REFERENCES

Curl WW. Popliteal cysts. Historical background and current knowledge. J Am Acad Orthop Surg 1996;4:129–133.

Rupp S, Seil R, Jochum P, Kohn D. Popliteal cysts in adults. Prevalence, associated intrarticular lesions, and results after arthroscopic treatment. Am J Sports Med 2002;30:112–115.

EXCISION OF LESION OF MENISCUS OR CAPSULE

CPT code   **27347** excision of lesion of meniscus or capsule (e.g., cyst, ganglion), knee

ICD-9 code   **717.5** meniscal cyst

INDICATIONS

- meniscal cyst or ganglion cyst causing functional or pain problems

ALTERNATIVE TREATMENTS

- observation
- activity modification
- aspiration, corticosteroid injections
- arthroscopy and intra-articular drainage of cyst with "opening" of cyst communication into intra-articular space

SURGICAL ANATOMY

Incision
- incision directly over cyst, lateral or medial

APPROACHES

Surgical Techniques
- excision in conjunction with open menisectomy or arthroscopic debridement
- incise to capsule and cyst
- complete removal of cyst
- remove damaged cartilage to stable rim if cyst etiology is secondary to meniscal pathology (most common)
- use intra-articular or intra-cystic injection of methylene blue, which may help identification and removal of cyst

POSTOPERATIVE MANAGEMENT

- crutches for safety
- pain medication as required
- DVT prophylaxis when indicated

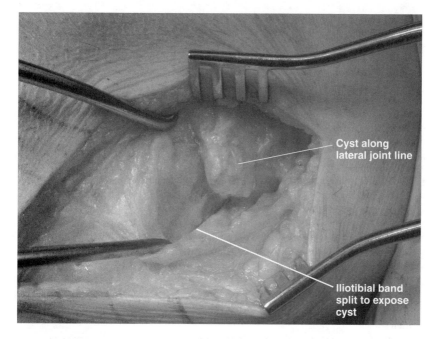

KNEE

Cyst along lateral joint line

Iliotibial band split to expose cyst

REHABILITATION

- ROM immediately to prevent stiffness
- strengthening once ROM re-established
- wean from crutches when gait normalized

COMPLICATIONS

- postoperative infection
- progression of arthritic changes
- exacerbation of arthritic condition (10%)
- recurrent cyst formation if incomplete excision

SELECTED REFERENCES

Reagan WD, McConkey JP, Loomer RL, Davidson RG. Cysts of the lateral meniscus: arthroscopy vs. arthroscopy plus open cystectomy. Arthroscopy 1989;5:274–281.

Hoppenfeld S, DeBoer P. Surgical exposures in orthopaedics: the anatomic approach. New York: JB Lippincott, 1984:395–420.

SUTURE OF INFRAPATELLAR TENDON, PRIMARY

CPT code   27380 suture of infrapatellar tendon, primary

ICD-9 code   727.66 rupture of patellar tendon

INDICATIONS

- rupture of patellar tendon with loss of active knee extension

ALTERNATIVE TREATMENTS

- nonoperative treatment for partial disruptions or in debilitated patients with neurologic conditions preventing ambulation and/or knee extensor ability in selected cases

SURGICAL ANATOMY

Incision
- midline incision from midpatella to tibial tubercle allowing exposure of retinaculum

APPROACHES

Surgical Techniques
- debride nonviable tendon tissue
- primary repair with nonabsorbable suture of tendon if cuff exists distal to patella
- nonabsorbable suture repair through drill holes in patella
- cerclage or nonabsorbable suture may be used to protect repair
- cerclage wire or suture placed through tunnel in patella and tibial tubercle
- suture retinaculum after joint wash-out and inspect articular injury

POSTOPERATIVE MANAGEMENT

- immobilizer with crutches
- partial weight bearing (PWB) for 4–6 weeks
- pain medication as needed

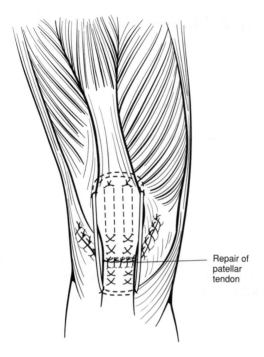

Repair of
patellar
tendon

REHABILITATION

- protected weight bearing in immobilizer
- protected, supervised ROM for 6 weeks
- quad sets, straight leg raising
- resume full function after 6 months

COMPLICATIONS

- re-rupture
- infection
- loss of knee extension strength

SELECTED REFERENCES

Matava MJ. Patellar tendon ruptures. J Am Acad Orthop Surg 199;4:287–296.
Marder RA, Timmerman LA. Primary repair of patellar tendon rupture without
augmentation. Am J Sports Med 1999;27:304–307.

SUTURE OF INFRAPATELLAR TENDON, SECONDARY RECONSTRUCTION

CPT code   27381 suture of infrapatellar tendon, secondary reconstruction, including fascial or tendon graft

ICD-9 code   727.66 patellar tendon rupture

INDICATIONS

- disruption of extensor mechanism at patellar tendon, delayed with poor tissue

ALTERNATIVE TREATMENTS

- nonoperative treatment for partial disruptions or in debilitated patients with neurologic conditions preventing ambulation and/or knee extensor ability in selected cases

SURGICAL ANATOMY

Incision
- midline incision from midpatella to tibial tubercle allowing exposure of retinaculum

APPROACHES

Surgical Techniques
- extend incision as necessary for harvesting of graft if augmentation required (e.g., hamstrings)
- debridement of nonviable tendon tissue
- primary repair with nonabsorbable suture of tendon if cuff exists and tendon gap less than 1 cm
- graft (semitendinosus [ST] or allograft) harvested and left attached to insertion
- semitendinosus tendon passed through tibial tunnel at tubercle and then through patella
- ST then reflected back along tendon and sutured to itself and remaining portion of distal patellar tendon
- use cerclage wire (needs to be removed in second procedure) or nonabsorbable suture
- cerclage wire or suture placed through tunnel in patella and tibial tubercle
- suture retinaculum after joint inspected and irrigated

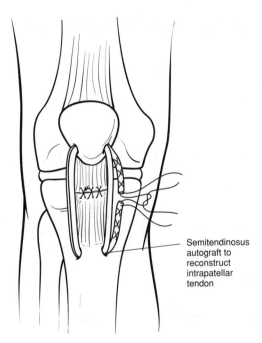

Semitendinosus autograft to reconstruct intrapatellar tendon

POSTOPERATIVE MANAGEMENT

- immobilizer with crutches for 2 weeks
- pain medication as needed

REHABILITATION

- protected weight bearing in immobilizer for 6–8 weeks
- advance ROM exercises to level determined in OR
- advance activity as tolerated initially in brace and then out of brace after 9 weeks or removal of cerclage (or both)

COMPLICATIONS

- re-rupture, extension weakness
- infection

SELECTED REFERENCES

McNally PD, Marcelli EA. Achilles allograft reconstruction of a chronic patellar tendon rupture. Arthroscopy 1998;14:340–344.
Larson RV, Simonian PT. Semitendinosus augmentation of acute patellar tendon repair with immediate immobilization. Am J Sports Med 1995;23:82–86.

SUTURE OF QUADRICEPS TENDON, PRIMARY

CPT code   27385 suture of quadriceps tendon, primary

ICD-9 code   727.65 quadriceps tendon rupture

INDICATION

- disruption of extensor mechanism of quadriceps insertion

ALTERNATIVE TREATMENTS

- nonoperative treatment for partial disruptions or in debilitated patients with neurologic conditions preventing ambulation and/or knee extensor ability in selected cases

SURGICAL ANATOMY

Incision
- midline incision from midthigh to midpatella

APPROACHES

Surgical Techniques
- debride nonviable tendon tissue
- primary repair with nonabsorbable suture (no. 2 or no. 5) of tendon if cuff exists proximal to patella
- if avulsed from patella, use nonabsorbable suture repair through longitudinal drill holes in patella
- suture placement in locking fashion to limit slippage (Krackow-Thomas suture technique)
- suture of retinaculum after intra-articular inspection and irrigation

POSTOPERATIVE MANAGEMENT

- immobilizer with crutches
- pain medication as needed

REHABILITATION

- protected weight bearing in immobilizer for 6 weeks
- advance ROM exercises to level determined in OR
- advance activity as tolerated initially in brace, and then out of brace after 6 weeks

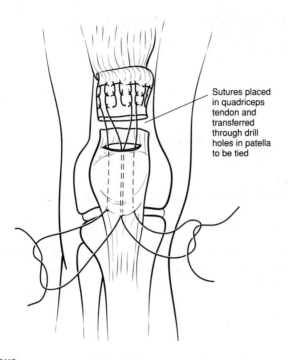

Sutures placed in quadriceps tendon and transferred through drill holes in patella to be tied

COMPLICATIONS

- re-rupture
- infection
- loss of knee extension and strength

SELECTED REFERENCES

O'Shea K, Kenny P, Donovan J, Condon F, McElwain JP. Outcomes following quadriceps tendon ruptures. Injury 2000;33:257–260.
Phillips B. Traumatic disorders. In: Crenshaw AH, ed. Campbell's operative orthopaedics, 8th ed. St. Louis: CV Mosby, 1992:1917–1919.

NOTES

_____
_____
_____
_____
_____
_____
_____

SUTURE OF QUADRICEPS TENDON, SECONDARY RECONSTRUCTION

CPT code   27386   suture of quadriceps tendon, secondary reconstruction, including fascial or tendon graft

ICD-9 code   727.65   rupture of quadriceps tendon

INDICATION

- disruption of extensor mechanism at quadriceps tendon

ALTERNATIVE TREATMENTS

- nonoperative treatment for partial disruptions or in debilitated patients with neurologic conditions preventing ambulation and/or knee extensor ability in selected cases

SURGICAL ANATOMY

Incision
- midline incision from distal thigh to midpatellar line allowing exposure of retinaculum

APPROACHES

Surgical Techniques
- extend incision as necessary for harvesting of graft (e.g., hamstrings) and for needed exposure
- debride nonviable tendon tissue
- primary repair with nonabsorbable suture of tendon, if cuff exists, and tendon gap less than 1 cm
- graft (semitendinosus or allograft) harvested as necessary, or exposure of superficial quadriceps fascial sheath for "turn-down" graft with "V-Y" advancement (see Illustration)
- reinforcement with free tendon graft or turned-down quadriceps
- graft placed through drill holes in patella
- suture retinaculum after joint inspected and irrigated

POSTOPERATIVE MANAGEMENT

- immobilizer with crutches for 6 weeks
- pain medication as needed

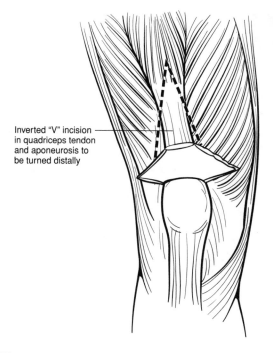

Inverted "V" incision in quadriceps tendon and aponeurosis to be turned distally

REHABILITATION

- protected weight bearing in immobilizer for 6 weeks
- advance ROM exercises to level determined in operating room to degree of flexion where repair was not under tension
- advance activity as tolerated initially in brace, and then out of brace after 9 weeks

COMPLICATIONS

- re-rupture
- infection
- loss of knee motion, quadriceps strength

SELECTED REFERENCES

Yilmaz C, Binnet MS, Narman S. Tendon lengthening repair and early mobilization in treatment of neglected bilateral simultaneous traumatic rupture of the quadriceps tendon. Knee Surg Sports Traumatol Arthrosc 2001;9:163–166.

Phillips B. Traumatic disorders. In: Crenshaw AH, ed. Campbell's operative orthopaedics, 8th ed. St. Louis: CV Mosby, 1992:1917–1921.

ARTHROTOMY WITH MENISCUS REPAIR

CPT code	27403 arthrotomy with meniscus repair, knee

ICD-9 codes	836.0 torn medial
	836.1 torn lateral meniscus

INDICATION

* unstable meniscal tear in the vascular zone

ALTERNATIVE TREATMENTS

* observation
* conservative care including activity modification, physical therapy, and anti-inflammatory medications
* arthroscopic meniscus repair

SURGICAL ANATOMY/APPROACHES

* appropriate posteromedial or posterolateral approach

Surgical Techniques/Incisions
Medial:

* incision 3 cm long, 2 cm below joint line
* incise pes fascia and retract medially
* incision through capsule will then allow direct access
* place 3–5 vertical sutures for repair

Lateral:

* posterolateral skin incision
* split posterior border of iliotibial band and biceps interval
* separate lateral gastrocnemius tendon from capsule
* vertical capsulotomy, repair tear as described previously

POSTOPERATIVE MANAGEMENT

* protect repair from shear forces for 6 weeks
* pain medication as needed

REHABILITATION

* protected weight bearing during healing phases
* crutches for 2–6 weeks
* advance activity slowly and then as tolerated after 6 weeks

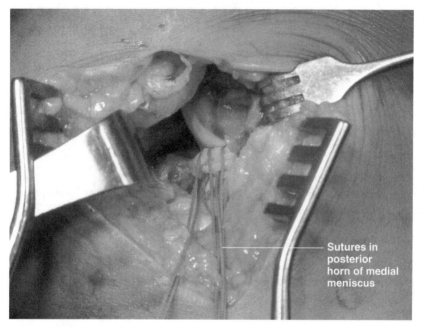

Sutures in posterior horn of medial meniscus

KNEE

COMPLICATIONS

- re-tear
- infection
- knee stiffness and adhesions
- nerve injury during approach

SELECTED REFERENCES

Rockborn P, Gillquist J. Results of open meniscal repair. Long-term follow-up study with matched uninjured controls. J Bone Joint Surg Br 2000;82:494–498.

DeHaven KE, Lohrer WA, Lovelock JE. Long-term results of open meniscal repair. Am J Sports Med 1995;23:524–530.

NOTES

REPAIR OF TORN COLLATERAL LIGAMENT

CPT code   **27405** arthrotomy, repair, primary, torn ligament and/or capsule, knee, collateral

ICD-9 codes   **844.0** lateral collateral ligament (LCL)
844.1 medial collateral ligament

INDICATIONS

• acute ligamentous injury
• acute capsular sprain, especially when associated with other ligamentous or meniscal injuries

ALTERNATIVE TREATMENTS

• observation
• conservative care including activity modification, physical therapy, and anti-inflammatory care
• open ligamentous reconstruction with autograft or allograft tissue

SURGICAL ANATOMY

Incision
• directly over lateral or medial collateral ligament

APPROACHES

Surgical Techniques
• dissection laterally is first through iliotibial band splitting fibers, the biceps femoris is then located and retracted posteriorly to protect peroneal nerve, nerve should be isolated and retracted itself when reconstruction on fibular head required (ITB can be taken off with bone from Gerdy's tubercle if more extensive dissection is necessary)
• direct repair possible if bony avulsion occurs or if isolated rupture without attenuation occurs
• attach avulsed ligament at origin or insertion
• suture anchors, staple, soft tissue screw
• midsubstance tears can have direct repair but may need augmentation with free-tendon graft
• free grafts must be securely fixed in bone tunnels or into blind bone tunnels with interference screws

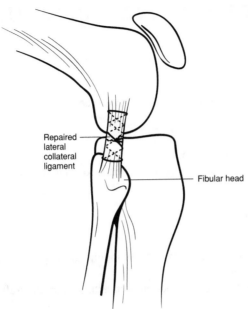

Repaired lateral collateral ligament

Fibular head

POSTOPERATIVE MANAGEMENT

- hold knee short of full extension for 1 week
- pain medication as needed

REHABILITATION

- crutches for 6–8 weeks
- begin active-assisted ROM between 10° and 45° at 1 week postoperatively and advance slowly to 90°
- hinged knee-brace to protect varus–valgus forces
- weight bearing when muscle strength sufficient to protect knee from rotational deforming forces

COMPLICATIONS

- re-tear or attenuation
- infection
- knee stiffness/adhesions
- nerve injury during approach

SELECTED REFERENCES

Krukhaug Y, Molster A, Rodt A, Strand T. Lateral ligament injuries of the knee. Knee Surg Sports Traumatol Arthrosc 1998;6:21–25.

Chen FS, Rokito AS, Pitman MI. Acute and chronic posterolateral rotatory instability of the knee. J Am Acad Orthop Surg 2000;8:97–110.

REPAIR OF MEDIAL COLLATERAL LIGAMENT

CPT code   27405   arthrotomy, repair, primary, torn ligament and/or capsule, knee, collateral

ICD-9 code   844.1   torn medial collateral ligament (MCL)

INDICATIONS

- acute ligamentous injury
- acute capsular sprain, especially when associated with other ligamentous or meniscal injuries

ALTERNATIVE TREATMENTS

- observation
- conservative care including activity modification, physical therapy, and anti-inflammatory care
- open ligamentous reconstruction with autograft or allograft tissue

SURGICAL ANATOMY

Incision

- incision directly over medial collateral ligament (MCL) or with "hockey stick" from adductor tubercle to medial tibial tubercle

APPROACHES

Surgical Techniques

- dissection medially is over MCL, which inserts up to 6 cm below joint line
- pes tendons and semimembranosus must be isolated
- direct repair is possible with no. 2 suture;
- if bony avulsion occurs, attach avulsed ligament at origin or insert with suture anchors, soft tissue staple, or screw/washer
- may be augmented with hamstring (see Illustration)

POSTOPERATIVE MANAGEMENT

- hold knee short of full extension for 1 week
- pain medication as needed

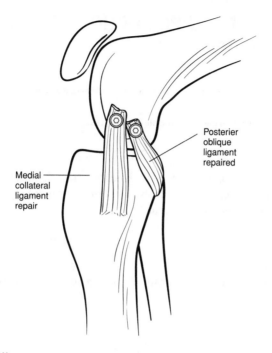

Posterier oblique ligament repaired

Medial collateral ligament repair

REHABILITATION

- crutches for 6–8 weeks
- begin active-assisted ROM between 10° and 45° at 1 week postoperatively, and advance slowly to 90°
- use hinged knee brace to protect varus–valgus forces
- weight bearing when muscle strength sufficient to protect knee from rotational deforming forces

COMPLICATIONS

- re-tear or attenuation
- infection
- knee stiffness/adhesions
- nerve injury during approach

SELECTED REFERENCES

Feagin JA. O'Donohue's triad. In: Feagin JA, ed. The crucial ligaments, 2nd ed. Churchill-Livingstone, 1994:39–53.

Muller W. The knee. Form, function and ligament reconstruction. New York: Springer-Verlag, 1983.

REPAIR OF TORN POSTERIOR CRUCIATE LIGAMENT

CPT code   **27407**   arthrotomy, repair, primary, torn ligament and/or capsule, knee, cruciate

ICD-9 code   **844.8**   torn posterior cruciate ligament (PCL)

INDICATIONS

- acute ligamentous injury, especially when multiple ligament injury occurs with capsular disruption (i.e., unable to perform arthroscopy)—rarely procedure of choice for ACL repairs

ALTERNATIVE TREATMENTS

- observation
- arthroscopic ligamentous reconstruction with autograft or allograft tissue

APPROACHES

Surgical Techniques

- direct anterior and/or posterior approach
- medial parapatellar-tendon retinacular incision to allow patellar translation or eversion

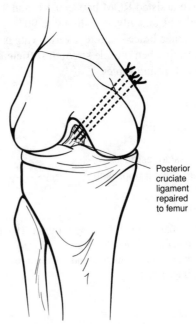

Posterior cruciate ligament repaired to femur

SURGICAL ANATOMY

Incision

- Krackow-Thomas or locking stitch placed into ligament stump
- femoral detachment: drill two, parallel 3.2 mm tunnels from medial femoral cortex near epicondyle into anatomic site in notch if tear close to femur
- use suture passer to retrieve sutures placed into ligament, pass to medial cortex and tension, and tie at 30° flexion with anterior force on knee
- if tear close to tibial attachment, drill-holes will be placed from anterior tibia posterior, sutures retrieved and passed to anterior and sutures tied on tibial cortex

KNEE

POSTOPERATIVE MANAGEMENT

- hold knee short of full extension for 4 weeks
- pain medication as needed

REHABILITATION

- crutches for 8 weeks
- begin active-assisted ROM between 10° and 45° at 1 week postoperatively, advance slowly to from 0 to 90° as tolerated
- weight bearing when muscle strength sufficient to protect knee from rotational deforming forces

COMPLICATIONS

- recurrent instability
- infection
- knee stiffness/adhesions
- nerve injury during approach

SELECTED REFERENCES

Ibrahim SA. Primary repair of the cruciate and collateral ligaments after traumatic dislocation of the knee. J Bone Joint Surg Br 1999;8:987–990.

Phillips B. Traumatic disorders. In: Crenshaw AH, ed. Campbell's operative orthopaedics, 8th ed. St. Louis: CV Mosby, 1992:1582–1586.

REPAIR OF TORN ANTERIOR OR POSTERIOR CRUCIATE LIGAMENT

CPT code   27407 arthrotomy, repair, primary, torn ligament and/or capsule, knee, cruciate

ICD-9 codes   844.2 torn anterior cruciate ligament (ACL)

KNEE   844.8 torn posterior cruciate ligament (PCL)

INDICATIONS

- acute ligamentous injury, especially when multiple ligament injury occurs with capsular disruption (i.e., unable to perform arthroscopy)
- acute bony avulsion of ligament

ALTERNATIVE TREATMENTS

- observation
- arthroscopic ligamentous reconstruction with autograft or allograft tissue

SURGICAL ANATOMY

- direct anterior and/or posterior approach

Incision

- medial parapatellar tendon retinacular incision to allow patellar translation or eversion

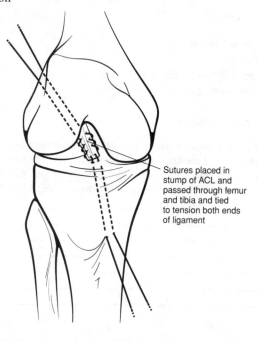

Sutures placed in stump of ACL and passed through femur and tibia and tied to tension both ends of ligament

APPROACHES

Surgical Techniques

- Krackow-Thomas or locking stitch placed into ligament stump
- for ACL, drill two, parallel 3.2 mm tunnels from lateral femoral cortex into anatomic site in notch, if tear is close to femoral attachment
- use suture passer to retrieve sutures placed into ligament, pass to lateral cortex and tension, and tie at 30° flexion with posterior force on knee
- if tear is close to tibial attachment, drill-holes will be placed from tibia into joint and sutures tied on tibial cortex

KNEE

POSTOPERATIVE MANAGEMENT

- hold knee short of full extension for 1 week
- pain medication as needed

REHABILITATION

- crutches for 8 weeks
- begin ROM between 10° and 45° at 1 week postoperatively, and advance slowly from 0 to 90° as tolerated
- weight bearing when muscle strength is sufficient to protect knee from rotational deforming forces

COMPLICATIONS

- re-tear or attenuation
- infection
- knee stiffness/adhesions
- nerve injury during approach

SELECTED REFERENCES

Steadman JR, Rodkey WG. Role of primary anterior cruciate ligament repair with or without augmentation. Clin Sports Med 1993;12:685–695.

Marshall JL, Warren RF, Wickiewicz TL, et al. The anterior cruciate ligament: a technique of repair and reconstruction. Clin Orthop 1979;143:97–106.

NOTES

_____

_____

_____

_____

_____

_____

_____

REPAIR OF TORN LIGAMENTS, COLLATERAL AND CRUCIATE

CPT code	27409 arthrotomy, repair, primary, torn ligament and/or capsule, knee, collateral and cruciate
ICD-9 code	844.0 torn lateral collateral ligament
	844.1 torn medial collateral ligament
	844.2 torn anterior cruciate ligament
	844.8 torn posterior cruciate ligament

INDICATIONS

- acute ligamentous injury, especially when multiple ligament injury occurs, i.e., knee dislocation
- acute bony avulsion of ligament

ALTERNATIVE TREATMENTS

- observation
- ligamentous reconstruction with autograft or allograft tissue of collateral ligament injuries with delayed ACL, posterior cruciate ligament (PCL) reconstructions

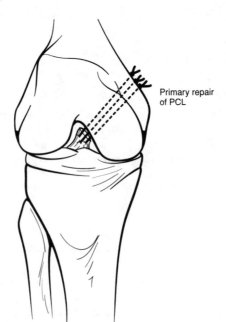

Primary repair of PCL

APPROACHES

- direct anterior and/or posterior approach

Surgical Incisions/Techniques

- medial parapatellar tendon retinacular incision to allow arthrotomy and patellar subluxation
- will permit exposure of tibial attachment of ACL, MCL, and femoral attachment of PCL
- posterior incision or posteromedial arthrotomy for tibial attachment of PCL
- approach to ACL femoral origin: can be from "outside-in," from lateral aspect of distal thigh; or from "inside-out," from anterior arthrotomy
- lateral incision for exposure of LCL and posterolateral corner
- incision laterally from proximal to lateral epicondyle along iliotibial band to a point midway between Gerdy's tubercle and the fibular head
- fascial incisions in IT band and inferior to biceps femoris to expose lateral structures and protect peroneal nerve
- harvest and prepare tendon grafts (autograft or allograft)
- locate anatomic origin and insertion points of ligaments to reconstruct
- create appropriate-sized bone tunnels
- pass cruciate grafts and fix on femur
- repair MCL, LCL, and/or posterolateral corner
- PCL must be fixed with knee at 90°
- ACL tibial fixation is done last

KNEE

POSTOPERATIVE MANAGEMENT

- hold knee short of full extension for 1 week
- pain medication as needed

REHABILITATION

- crutches for 8 weeks
- begin active-assisted ROM between 10° and 45° at 1 week postoperatively and advance slowly to from 0 to 90°
- brace in full extension for 4 weeks if collateral repairs done simultaneously
- weight bearing when muscle strength sufficient to protect knee from rotational deforming forces

COMPLICATIONS

- recurrent instability
- infection
- knee stiffness/adhesions
- neurovascular injury during approach

SELECTED REFERENCES

Ibrahim SA. Primary repair of the cruciate and collateral ligaments after traumatic dislocation of the knee. J Bone Joint Surg Br 1999;81:987–990.

Phillips B. Traumatic disorders. In: Crenshaw AH, ed. Campbell's operative orthopaedics, 8th ed. St. Louis: CV Mosby, 1992:1582–1586.

NOTES

_____
_____
_____
_____
_____
_____
_____
_____
_____
_____

KNEE

TIBIAL TUBERCLE OSTEOTOMY

CPT code   27418 anterior tibial tubercleplasty (e.g., Maquet type procedure)

ICD-9 code   715.96 knee osteoarthritis

                    718.36 internal derangement

INDICATIONS

- recurrent subluxations and/or dislocations of patella
- significant patellofemoral arthrosis or chondral irregularity

ALTERNATIVE TREATMENTS

- observation and conservative physical therapy
- arthroscopic debridement, chondroplasty, soft tissue realignment

APPROACHES

Surgical Techniques

- direct anterior approach with slight proximal deviation to lateral aspect of patella
- dissection of anterior compartment periosteally from lateral tibial face
- dissection of tubercle medially to identify patellar tendon insertion clearly
- osteotomize tubercle in traditional horizontal fashion or obliquely as in Fulkerson osteotomy technique
- protect anterior tibial artery with Homan retractor
- obtain tricortical iliac crest graft if necessary to anteriorize tubercle
- secure with two bicortical screws
- perform lateral release to extent necessary to avoid iatrogenic patellar tilt

POSTOPERATIVE MANAGEMENT

- hold knee in full extension for 1 week
- pain medication as needed

REHABILITATION

- begin quadriceps sets and straight leg raises immediately after surgery
- patellar mobilization and flexion without resistance to begin 1 week postoperatively
- partial or protected weight bearing for 4–6 weeks
- immobilizer and crutches until osteotomy heals

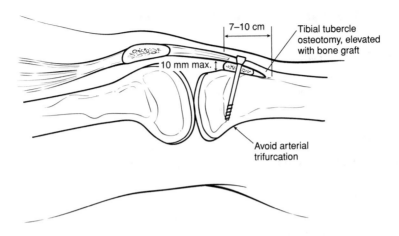

7–10 cm

Tibial tubercle
osteotomy, elevated
with bone graft

10 mm max.

Avoid arterial
trifurcation

KNEE

COMPLICATIONS

- infection
- tibial fracture, skin necrosis

SELECTED REFERENCES

Fulkerson JP, Becker GJ, Meaney JA, Miranda M, Folcik MA. Anteromedial tibial
    tubercle transfer without bone graft. Am J Sports Med 1990;18:490–496.
Rappoport LH, Browne MG, Wickiewicz TL. The Maquet osteotomy. Orthop Clin
    North Am 1992;23:645–656.

NOTES

REPAIR OF PATELLAR DISLOCATION

CPT code   27420 reconstruction of dislocating patella (e.g., Hauser type procedure)

ICD-9 code   755.69 subluxing patella
                    836.3 dislocating patella

INDICATIONS

- recurrent subluxations and/or dislocations of patella

ALTERNATIVE TREATMENTS

- observation and conservative physical therapy
- bracing, activity modification

APPROACHES

Surgical Techniques

- direct anterior approach with slight proximal deviation to lateral aspect of patella
- dissection of anterior compartment periosteally from lateral tibial face
- dissection of tubercle medially to identify patellar tendon insertion clearly
- osteotomize tubercle, horizontal or oblique
- protect anterior tibial artery with Homan retractor
- shift tubercle medially and distally
- secure with two, bicortical screws
- perform lateral release
- adjust medialization of tubercle to center patellar tracking

POSTOPERATIVE MANAGEMENT

- immobilization in extension
- pain medication as needed

REHABILITATION

- begin quadriceps sets and straight leg raises immediately after surgery
- patellar mobilization and flexion
- protected weight bearing for 4–6 weeks
- immobilizer and crutches until osteotomy heals

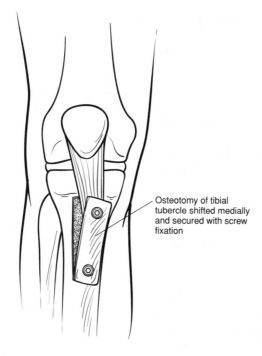

Osteotomy of tibial tubercle shifted medially and secured with screw fixation

KNEE

COMPLICATIONS

- iatrogenic medial instability
- infection
- recurrent instability
- loss of motion, arthritis

SELECTED REFERENCES

Naranja RJ, Reilly PJ, Kuhlman JR, Haut E, Torg JS. Long-term evaluation of the Elmslie-Trillat-Maquet procedure for patellofemoral dysfunction. Am J Sports Med 1996;24:779–784.

Rillman P, Dutly A, Kieser C, Berbig R. Modified Elmslie-Trillat procedure for instability of the patella. Knee Surg Sports Traumatol Arthrosc 1998;6:31–35.

NOTES

_____

_____

_____

_____

_____

_____

REPAIR OF PATELLAR DISLOCATION, EXTENSOR ALIGNMENT

CPT code   27422   reconstruction of dislocating patella (e.g., Hauser type procedure) with extensor realignment and/or muscle advancement or release (e.g., Campbell, Goldwaite type procedure)

ICD-9 code   755.69   subluxing patella
                 836.3   dislocating patella

INDICATIONS

* recurrent subluxations and/or dislocations of patella, especially in skeletally immature individuals

ALTERNATIVE TREATMENTS

* observation and conservative physical therapy
* bracing, activity modification
* isolated tibial tubercle osteotomy
* arthroscopic proximal realignment

APPROACHES

Surgical Techniques

* anterior peripatellar approach
* dissection of tubercle medially and laterally
* expose quadriceps (vastus medialis obliquus [VMO]) attachment to superior and medial patella and/or patellar tendon attachment to patella and tubercle, depending on choice of realignment procedure (proximal or distal)
* take off VMO from 12 o'clock to 3 o'clock for left knee, including 2–3 cm split up quad tendon and 2-cm down medial retinaculum
* advance VMO onto patella approximately 5 mm or to appropriate tension; tie down with suture anchors or periosteal stitches and quad tendon/retinacular repair
* osteotomize tibial tubercle and shift medially, fixation with screws or staple

POSTOPERATIVE MANAGEMENT

* hold knee in full extension for 1 week
* pain medication as needed

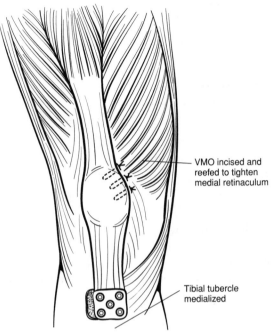

VMO incised and
reefed to tighten
medial retinaculum

Tibial tubercle
medialized

REHABILITATION

- quadriceps sets, straight leg raising (SLR), patellar mobilization
- supervised ROM
- partial weight bearing for 4–6 weeks
- immobilizer and crutches until osteotomy heals, if osteotomy performed

COMPLICATIONS

- iatrogenic medial instability
- infection
- recurrent instability

SELECTED REFERENCES

Scuderi G, Cuomo F, Scott WN. Lateral release and proximal realignment for patellar
  subluxation and dislocation. A long-term follow-up. J Bone Joint Surg Am
  1988;70:856–861.
Myers P, Williams A, Dodds R, Bulow J. The three-in-one proximal and distal soft
  tissue patellar realignment procedure: results, and its place in the management
  of patellofemoral instability. Am J Sports Med 1999;27:575–579.

LATERAL RETINACULAR RELEASE

CPT code	**27425** lateral retinacular release

ICD-9 code	**718.36** internal derangement
	755.69 subluxation of patella

INDICATIONS

- excessive lateral pressure syndrome
- lateral patellar tilt

ALTERNATIVE TREATMENTS

- observation, physical therapy
- bracing, activity modification
- arthroscopic release
- tibial tubercle osteotomy or soft tissue realignment procedure

SURGICAL ANATOMY

Incision

- small (3–4 cm) incision directly over lateral retinaculum
- short incision over retinaculum approximately 1 cm lateral to patella

APPROACHES

Surgical Techniques

- dissect down to retinaculum
- amount of release should not exceed vastus lateralis muscle proximally
- distally the patellar-tibial "ligament" must be incised (usually exists distal to lateral parapatellar tendon arthroscopy portal)

POSTOPERATIVE MANAGEMENT

- compressive dressing for 3–4 days with direct compression of lateral retinaculum (i.e., rolled-up Kerlex)
- pain medication as needed

REHABILITATION

- begin quadriceps sets and straight leg raises immediately
- patellar mobilization, ROM, and effusion reduction to begin postoperative week 1
- return to athletic activities once quadriceps strength at or near normal

KNEE

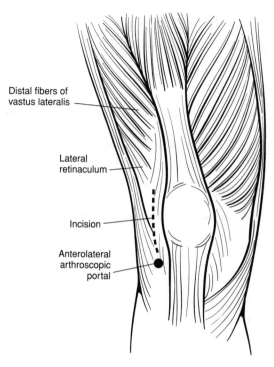

Distal fibers of vastus lateralis

Lateral retinaculum

Incision

Anterolateral arthroscopic portal

COMPLICATIONS

- iatrogenic medial instability
- infection
- hematoma

SELECTED REFERENCES

Fulkerson JP. Diagnosis and treatment of patients with patellofemoral pain. Am J Sports Med 2002;3:447–456.
O'Neill DB. Open lateral retinacular lengthening compared with arthroscopic release. A prospective, randomized outcome study. J Bone Joint Surg Am 1997;79:95–100.

NOTES

LIGAMENTOUS RECONSTRUCTION, KNEE, EXTRA-ARTICULAR, MEDIAL COLLATERAL

CPT code	27427 ligamentous reconstruction (augmentation), knee; extra-articular
ICD-9 code	844.0/844.1/844.2/844.8 chronic cruciate deficiency or chronic collateral ligament deficiency

INDICATIONS

- acute or chronic ligamentous deficiency involving MCL complex
- combined instability pattern, usually with ACL or PCL (or both) deficiency

ALTERNATIVE TREATMENTS

- observation, physical therapy
- bracing, activity modification
- other graft sources: semitendinosus; quadriceps
- delayed primary repair (seldom indicated; requires good tissue quality)

APPROACHES

Surgical Techniques

- most often procedure performed in conjunction with CPT codes 29888, 29889, 27407, 27428
- MCL—using Achilles allograft
- anteromedial "hockey stick" incision
- expose MCL complex, superficial, deep MCL, posterior oblique ligament, posteromedial capsule
- expose epicondyle and distal attachment of MCL, 12 cm below joint line
- use K-wire and suture to evaluate isometric points through range of motion
- prepare Achilles allograft into quadrangular shape
- pass graft and fix with interference screw, ligament button, staple, or screw/washer, etc., on femur first and then on tibia
- reef posterior capsule and posterior oblique ligament (POL) to MCL construct

POSTOPERATIVE MANAGEMENT

- crutches, brace for 6–8 weeks
- pain medication as needed

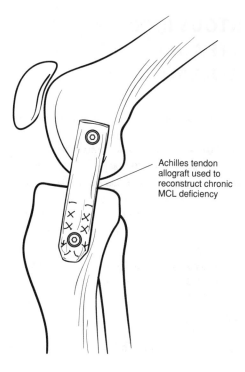

Achilles tendon
allograft used to
reconstruct chronic
MCL deficiency

REHABILITATION

- touch-down weight bearing for 6 weeks
- restricted ROM for 4–6 weeks
- quadriceps rehabilitation; delay hamstrings for 3–4 months

COMPLICATIONS

- failure, attenuation
- infection
- neurovascular injury

SELECTED REFERENCES

Larson RV, Metcalf MH. Posterior cruciate ligament reconstruction: associated
    extraarticular procedures medial and lateral. Tech Orthop 2001;16:148–156.
Borden PS, Kantaras AT, Caborn DN. Medial collateral ligament reconstruction with
    allograft using double-bundle technique. Arthroscopy 2002;18:E19.

LIGAMENTOUS RECONSTRUCTION, KNEE, EXTRA-ARTICULAR, LATERAL COLLATERAL; POSTEROLATERAL COMPLEX

CPT code   **27427** ligamentous reconstruction (augmentation), knee; extra-articular

ICD-9 code   **844.0** lateral collateral ligament (LCL) deficiency

844.1 chronic medial collateral ligament (MCL) deficiency

844.2 chronic anterior/posterior cruciate ligament deficiency

INDICATIONS

- acute or chronic ligamentous deficiency involving posterolateral ligament complex (LCL, popliteal muscle)
- combined instability pattern usually with ACL or PCL (or both) deficiency

ALTERNATIVE TREATMENTS

- observation, physical therapy, bracing, activity modification
- biceps tenodesis, BTB, or Achilles allograft
- delayed primary repair (seldom indicated, requires good tissue quality)

APPROACHES

Surgical Techniques

- most often procedure performed in conjunction with CPT codes 29888, 29889, 27407, 27428
- posterolateral—using semitendinosus
- incision lateral "hockey stick," ending between Gerdy's tubercle and fibular head
- expose iliotibial (IT) band, biceps femoris
- fascial incision posterior to biceps femoris to isolate and protect peroneal nerve
- second fascial incision between IT band and biceps femoris
- retract lateral gastrocnemius tendon muscle to expose posterolateral corner
- third fascial incision over epicondyle to identify LCL origin and trace to fibular styloid
- make posterolateral arthrotomy posterior to LCL
- expose popliteal tendon and attachment to lateral condyle
- drill 6–7 mm, anterior to posterior in fibular head
- find isometric position with K-wire on lateral femoral epicondyle
- pass graft and fix with interference screw, ligament button, staple, screw/washer, etc.

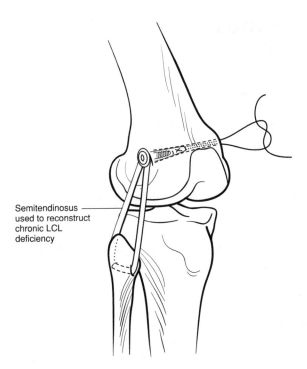

Semitendinosus used to reconstruct chronic LCL deficiency

KNEE

POSTOPERATIVE MANAGEMENT

- crutches, brace for 6–8 weeks
- pain medication as needed

REHABILITATION

- touch-down weight bearing for 6 weeks
- restricted ROM for 4–6 weeks
- quadriceps rehabilitation; delay hamstrings for 3–4 months

COMPLICATIONS

- failure, attenuation
- infection
- neurovascular injury

SELECTED REFERENCES

Larson RV, Metcalf MH. Posterior cruciate ligament reconstruction: associated extraarticular procedures medial and lateral. Tech Orthop 2001;16:148–156.
Fanelli GC, Larson RV. Practical management of posterolateral instability of the knee. Arthroscopy 2002;18(2 Suppl 1):1–8.

LIGAMENTOUS RECONSTRUCTION, KNEE, INTRA-ARTICULAR

CPT code   27428 ligamentous reconstruction, knee; intra-articular

ICD-9 code   844.2 torn anterior cruciate ligament

INDICATIONS

- acute ligamentous disruption
- chronic ligamentous attenuation with instability

ALTERNATIVE TREATMENTS

- observation, physical therapy, bracing, activity modification
- arthroscopic intra-articular reconstruction

APPROACHES

Surgical Techniques

- anterior parapatellar approach, anteromedial
- arthrotomy, or expose through patellar tendon defect after graft harvest
- debride ligament stumps
- perform notchplasty, prepare tibial tunnel with guide wire from anteromedial tibial cortex into tibial stump
- create femoral tunnel from inside-out with knee hyperflexed with $\frac{3}{32}$-in. guide wire starting at femoral attachment exiting lateral cortex
- other option is to create femoral tunnel from lateral cortex outside-in after lateral incision along lateral epicondyle
- harvest graft (patellar tendon, hamstring, or quadriceps tendon) and size diameter
- drill appropriate tunnels, usually 8–11 mm
- pass graft and fix with interference screw, ligament button, staple, screw/washer, etc.

POSTOPERATIVE MANAGEMENT

- crutches, brace as needed
- pain medication as needed

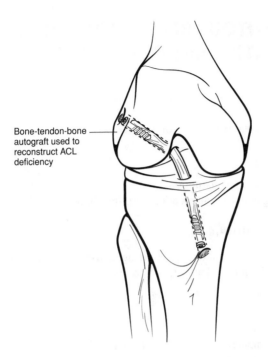

Bone-tendon-bone autograft used to reconstruct ACL deficiency

REHABILITATION

- partial weight bearing for 2–3 weeks
- ROM immediately
- work to gain extension for ACL and flexion for PCL early

COMPLICATIONS

- failure, attenuation
- infection
- neurovascular injury

SELECTED REFERENCES

Lambert KL, Cunningham RR. Open ACL reconstruction with patellar tendon and interference screw fixation. In: Feagin JA, ed. The crucial ligaments, 2nd ed. New York: Churchill-Livingstone, 1994:521–526.

Shelbourne KD, Gray T. Anterior cruciate ligament reconstruction with autogenous patellar tendon graft followed by accelerated rehabilitation. A two-to-nine year follow up. Am J Sports Med 1997;25:786–795.

LIGAMENTOUS RECONSTRUCTION, KNEE, INTRA-ARTICULAR (OPEN)

CPT code   **27428** ligamentous reconstruction, knee; intra-articular

ICD-9 code   **844.8** torn posterior cruciate ligament

INDICATIONS

- acute ligamentous disruption
- chronic ligamentous attenuation with instability

ALTERNATIVE TREATMENTS

- observation, physical therapy, bracing, activity modification
- arthroscopic intra-articular reconstruction

APPROACHES

Surgical Techniques
- anterior parapatellar approach, anteromedial
- arthrotomy, or expose through patellar tendon defect after graft harvest
- debride ligament stumps
- use posteromedial capsulotomy to access PCL tibial attachment site and protect popliteal neurovascular structures
- prepare tibial tunnel with guide wire from anteromedial tibial cortex into posterior tibial PCL attachment
- use image intensifier to monitor guide-pin
- create femoral tunnel from outside-in from medial femoral epicondylar region with guide wire placed at the 11 o'clock position for a left knee (1 o'clock for right), about 8–10 mm proximal to the articular edge within the intercondylar notch
- harvest graft (patellar tendon, hamstring, or quadriceps tendon) and size diameter
- drill appropriate tunnels usually 11–12 mm
- pass graft and fix with interference screw, ligament button, staple, screw/washer, etc.
- tension at 90° flexion with an anterior drawer applied

POSTOPERATIVE MANAGEMENT

- crutches, brace in extension
- pain medication as needed

KNEE

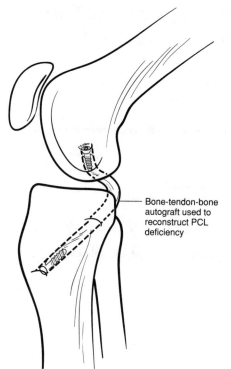

Bone-tendon-bone autograft used to reconstruct PCL deficiency

REHABILITATION

- partial weight bearing and immobilize in extension for 2–3 weeks
- limit flexion to 90° for first 6 weeks
- work to gain extension for ACL and flexion for PCL early

COMPLICATIONS

- failure, attenuation
- infection
- neurovascular injury

SELECTED REFERENCE

Sisk TD. Knee Injuries. In: Crenshaw AH, ed. Campbell's operative orthopaedics, 8th ed. St. Louis: CV Mosby, 1992:1691–1695.

OSTEOTOMY, PROXIMAL TIBIA, CLOSING WEDGE TECHNIQUE

CPT code	27457 osteotomy, proximal tibia, including fibular excision or osteotomy, after epiphyseal closure; closing wedge
ICD-9 code	715.96 arthritis, medial compartment of knee

INDICATIONS

- symptomatic genu varum
- medial compartment gonarthrosis

ALTERNATIVE TREATMENTS

- observation, orthotics with wedges, unloader braces
- opening wedge osteotomy
- hemicallotasis

SURGICAL ANATOMY

Incision

- midline incision
- anterolateral incisions

APPROACHES

- exposure of lateral tibia by reflecting anterior compartment posteriorly
- expose patellar insertion into tubercle and release more proximal fibers for visualization
- fibular shaft exposure through same incision or secondary incision directly below neck and peroneal nerve, or resect proximal tibulofibular joint

SURGICAL TECHNIQUES

- plan osteotomy angles preoperatively, and place guide pins using C-arm
- cut osteotomy using commercial guides, or free-hand, to desired level with care not to violate contralateral cortex or fracture into joint surface fracture
- check correction of mechanical axis using C-arm (hip to ankle)
- plate fixation with large cancellous screws proximally and bicortical screws distally
- close apposition of surfaces for closing wedge procedure with oblique fibular osteotomy below proximal tibulofibular joint indicated

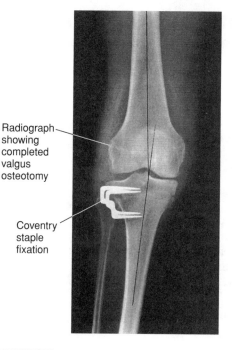

Radiograph showing completed valgus osteotomy

Coventry staple fixation

KNEE

POSTOPERATIVE MANAGEMENT

- crutches, non-weight-bearing
- pain medication as needed

REHABILITATION

- ROM immediately with quadriceps activation, patellar mobilization
- partial weight bearing with brace and crutches until healing occurs

COMPLICATIONS

- loss of correction
- fracture through contralateral cortex
- infection

SELECTED REFERENCES

Marti RK, Verhagen RA, Kerkhoffs GM, Moojen TM. Proximal tibial varus osteotomy. Indications, technique, and five to twenty-one-year results. J Bone Joint Surg Am 2001;83-A:164–170.

Fowler PJ, Tan JL, Brown GA. Medial opening wedge osteotomy. Op Tech Sports Med 2000;8:32–38.

OSTEOTOMY, PROXIMAL TIBIA, OPENING WEDGE TECHNIQUE

CPT code	27457 osteotomy, proximal tibia, including fibular excision or osteotomy, after epiphyseal closure
ICD-9 code	715.96 medial compartment arthritis

INDICATIONS

- symptomatic genu varum or valgum

ALTERNATIVE TREATMENTS

- observation, orthotics with wedges, unloader braces
- closing wedge osteotomy
- hemicallotasis

SURGICAL ANATOMY

Incision

- midline incision
- anteromedial incision over pes tendons
- expose pes anserine tendons medially, takedown of anterior MCL fibers as necessary
- expose patellar insertion into tubercle and release more proximal fibers for visualization

APPROACHES

Surgical Techniques

- plan osteotomy angles preoperatively and place guide pins using C-arm, 1.5–2.0 cm distal to joint line
- cut osteotomy using commercial guides or free-hand to desired level with care not to violate contralateral cortex or fracture into joint surface
- open osteotomy to desired correction and insert plate with two cancellous screws proximally and bicortical fixation distally
- opening wedge osteotomy bone-grafting with tricortical graft for large corrections, cancellous or allograft bone for smaller corrections

POSTOPERATIVE MANAGEMENT

- crutches, non-weight-bearing
- pain medication as needed

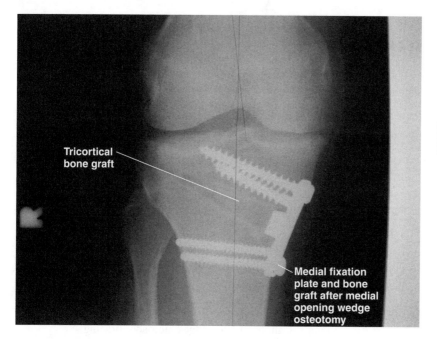

Tricortical bone graft

KNEE

Medial fixation plate and bone graft after medial opening wedge osteotomy

REHABILITATION

- ROM immediately with quadriceps activation and patellar mobilization
- partial weight bearing with brace and crutches for 6 weeks

COMPLICATIONS

- loss of correction
- fracture through contralateral cortex
- infection

SELECTED REFERENCES

Marti RK, Verhagen RA, Kerkhoffs GM, Moojen TM. Proximal tibial varus osteotomy. Indications, technique, and five to twenty-one-year results. J Bone Joint Surg Am 2001;83-A:164–170.

Fowler PJ, Tan JL, Brown GA. Medial opening wedge osteotomy. Op Tech Sports Med 2000;8:32–38.

AUTOLOGOUS CHONDROCYTE IMPLANTATION

CPT code	27599 unlisted procedure, knee, autologous chondrocyte implantation (Carticel) (plus code +1786)
ICD-9 code	715.96 osteoarthritis
	716.1 traumatic orthropathy
	717 internal derangement of knee
	732.7 osteochondritis dissecans of knee

INDICATION

- symptomatic chondral lesion greater than 2 cm^2
  (Note: Tibial tubercle osteotomy recommended for ALL trochlear procedures and for any condylar procedures with any malalignment of mechanical axis.)

ALTERNATIVE TREATMENTS

- observation, therapy, orthotics with wedges, unloader bracing
- arthroscopic chondroplasty, debridement, abrasion arthroplasty, microfracture

APPROACHES

- previous chondrocyte (cartilage) biopsy needed, usually done at index procedure arthroscopically
- implantation done open via midline incision, medial or lateral patellar arthrotomy with translation of patella to allow direct access and visualization of chondral defect
- trochlear lesions requiring tibial tubercle osteotomy should have lateral approach (release) with or without reflection of extensor mechanism for exposure

Incision/Surgical Techniques

- periosteal patch can be harvested through separate incision over anteromedial tibia or through midline incision from femoral condyles
- careful, meticulous debridement of loose, nonviable cartilage without creating any subchondral bleeding
- suturing of periosteal patch with no. 6 Vicryl and sealed with Tisseel™ or fibrin glue
- watertight testing with saline followed by introduction of cells and sealing of pouch
- osteotomies (proximal tibia or tibial tubercle) completed, or at least prepared prior to cell injection

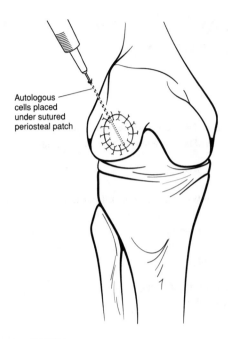

Autologous cells placed under sutured periosteal patch

POSTOPERATIVE MANAGEMENT

- crutches, non-weight-bearing
- continuous passive motion for 6 weeks to begin on postoperative day 1
- pain medication as needed

REHABILITATION

- effusion reduction, patellar mobilization, assisted-active ROM over first 3 weeks
- strengthening, partial weight bearing begins at week 4

COMPLICATIONS

- persistent pain or effusion (often until 3 months)
- infection
- delamination

SELECTED REFERENCES

Sgaglione NA, Miniaci A, Gillogly SD, Carter. Update on advanced surgical techniques in the treatment of traumatic focal articular cartilage lesions in the knee. Arthroscopy 2002;18(2 Suppl 1):9–32.

Brittberg M, Tallheden T, Sjogren-Jansson B, Lindahl A, Peterson L. Autologous chondrocytes for articular cartilage repair. Clin Orthop 2001;(391 Suppl):S337–348. Review.

MENISCUS ALLOGRAFT RECONSTRUCTION, KEYHOLE TECHNIQUE

CPT code   27599 knee, unlisted (meniscus allograft reconstruction, keyhole technique)

ICD-9 codes   836.0 tear of medial cartilage or meniscus of knee
                   836.1 tear of lateral cartilage or meniscus of knee

INDICATIONS

- meniscal deficiency without substantial chondral damage
- isolated medial-lateral compartment pain
- normal alignment, stable knee

ALTERNATIVE TREATMENTS

- activity modification, injections
- osteotomy or arthroplasty

APPROACHES

- standard knee arthroscopy, two or three portals

Incision

- posterolateral or posteromedial incisions for suture retrieval as per meniscal repair technique

Surgical Techniques

- systematic examination of entire intra-articular space
- excise and roughen meniscal-synovial rim to create bleeding base for increased allograft healing
- select and drill keyhole in proximal tibia along line of anterior and posterior roots of meniscus
- using template, sculpt meniscus into appropriate keyhole shape and advance and push meniscus into place with assistance of single strong (no. 2 or bigger) suture previously placed in meniscus and advanced through posteromedial or posterolateral corner
- secure meniscus with sutures through cannula placed across allograft synovial junction and tied sequentially against posterior capsule (accessory posteromedial or posterolateral skin incision required for repair of meniscus)

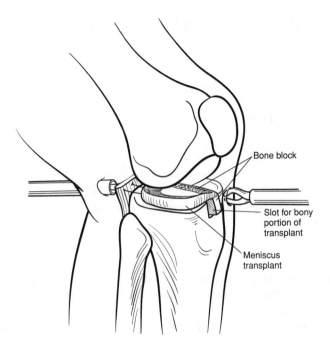

Bone block

Slot for bony
portion of
transplant

Meniscus
transplant

POSTOPERATIVE MANAGEMENT

- pain medication as needed
- crutches as needed

REHABILITATION

- effusion reduction, straight leg raises, quadriceps activation with knee in extension
- patellar mobilization
- minimal weight bearing for 6 weeks
- careful avoidance of axial compression with knee flexed greater than 90°

COMPLICATIONS

- stiffness and adhesions
- infection
- failure of repair (10–25%)

SELECTED REFERENCES

Rodeo SA. Meniscal allografts—where do we stand? Am J Sports Med 2001;29:246–261.
Rath E, Richmond JC, Yassir W, Albright JD, Gundogan F. Meniscal allograft transplantation: two eight- year results. Am J Sports Med 2001;29:410–414.

OSTEOCHONDRAL ALLOGRAFTING

CPT code   27599 unlisted procedure, knee
osteochondral allografting

ICD-9 code   715.96 osteoarthritis

INDICATIONS

*   symptomatic chondral lesion greater than 6 cm^2
    (Note: Tibial tubercle osteotomy should be considered for trochlear
    procedures and for condylar procedures with any malalignment of
    mechanical axis.)

ALTERNATIVE TREATMENTS

*   observation, therapy, orthotics with wedges, unloader bracing
*   arthroscopic chondroplasty, debridement, abrasion arthroplasty,
    microfracture
*   osteochondral autografting or autologous chondrocyte implantation
*   osteotomy

SURGICAL ANATOMY

Incision

*   open via midline incision, medial or lateral patellar arthrotomy
    with translation of patella to allow direct access and visualization
    of chondral defect

APPROACHES

*   trochlear lesions requiring tibial tubercle osteotomy should have lateral
    approach (release) with or without reflection of extensor mechanism
    for exposure

Surgical Techniques

*   harvest usually from proximal medial condyle
*   debridement defining of lesion
*   measure recipient site
*   measure and match contour of donor site
*   harvest, osteotomy may be indicated
*   graft fixation: press-fit or internal fixation

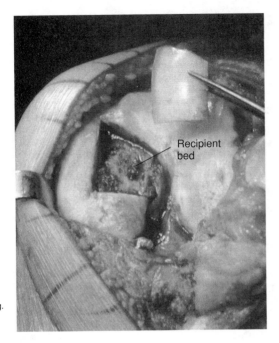

Recipient
bed

From Bugbee WD. Fresh
osteochondral allografting.
Op Tech Sports Med
2000;8:158, Figure 3.

POSTOPERATIVE MANAGEMENT

- crutches, non-weight-bearing
- consider continuous passive motion to begin postoperative day 1
- pain medication as needed

REHABILITATION

- effusion reduction, patellar mobilization, assisted-active ROM over first 3 weeks
- strengthening, partial weight bearing begins at 6 weeks or when incorporation evident

COMPLICATIONS

- persistent pain or effusion
- infection

SELECTED REFERENCES

Aubin PP, Cheah HK, Davis AM, Gross AE. Long-term follow-up of fresh femoral osteochondral allografts for posttraumatic knee defects. Clin Orthop 2001; (391 Suppl):S318–327.
Garrett JC. Fresh osteochondral allografts for treatment of articular defects in osteochondritis dissecans of the lateral femoral condyle in adults. Clin Orthop 1994;303:33–37.

OSTEOCHONDRAL AUTOGRAFTING

| CPT code | 27599 unlisted procedure, knee |
| | osteochondral autografting |

| ICD-9 code | 715.96 osteoarthritis |

INDICATIONS

- symptomatic chondral lesion less than 1 cm^2
  (Note: Tibial tubercle osteotomy should be considered for trochlear procedures and for condylar procedures with any malalignment of mechanical axis.)

ALTERNATIVE TREATMENTS

- observation, therapy, orthotics with wedges, unloader bracing
- arthroscopic chondroplasty, debridement, abrasion arthroplasty, microfracture

APPROACHES

- grafting performed arthroscopically or open
- arthroscopic approach sometimes aided by open osteochondral donor harvest
- open via midline incision, medial, or lateral patellar arthrotomy with translation of patella to allow direct access and visualization of chondral defect
- trochlear lesions requiring tibial tubercle osteotomy should have lateral approach (release) with or without reflection of extensor mechanism for exposure
- harvest usually from proximal lateral condyle

Surgical Techniques

- debridement and specific defining of lesion
- prepare recipient site with harvester
- obtain donor graft, stay perpendicular
- insert graft into recipient site
- osteotomies (proximal tibia or tibial tubercle) may be done simultaneously to correct alignment abnormalities

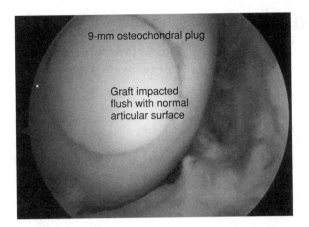

POSTOPERATIVE MANAGEMENT

- crutches, non-weight-bearing
- consider continuous passive motion, to begin on postoperative day 1
- pain medication as needed

REHABILITATION

- effusion reduction, patellar mobilization, and active-assisted ROM over first 3 weeks
- strengthening, partial weight bearing begins at week 4

COMPLICATIONS

- persistent pain or effusion
- infection

SELECTED REFERENCES

Buckwalter JA, Mankin HJ. Articular cartilage: degeneration, osteoarthritis, repair, regeneration, and transplantation. Instr Course Lect 1998;47:487–504. Review.
Bobic V. Autologous osteochondral grafts in the management of articular cartilage lesions. Orthopade 1999;28:19–25.

NOTES

ARTHROSCOPICALLY AIDED TREATMENT OF INTERCONDYLAR SPINE AND/OR TUBEROSITY FRACTURE OF KNEE WITHOUT FIXATION

CPT code   29850 arthroscopically aided treatment of intercondylar spine(s) and/or tuberosity fracture(s) of the knee, with or without manipulation; without internal or external fixation (includes arthroscopy)

ICD-9 code   823.00 fracture tibial eminence

INDICATIONS

• tibial avulsion fractures rendering ACL or PCL incompetent with displacement of fragment

ALTERNATIVE TREATMENTS

• observation, casting in extension
• arthroscopic reduction with fixation (CPT code, 29851)

APPROACHES

• knee arthroscopy using anterior-inferior lateral and medial portals with intra-articular manipulation of bone fragment into fracture base

Surgical Techniques

• removal of loose bony fragments (non-reparable) and lavage of the knee
• reduction of fracture fragment; usually reduction is blocked by intermeniscal ligament interposed between fragment and base

POSTOPERATIVE MANAGEMENT

• crutches, non-weight-bearing
• cast or immobilize with confirmation of reduction of fragment
• pain medication as needed

REHABILITATION

• effusion reduction, straight leg raises, and quadriceps activation with knee in extension
• begin ROM once fragment healed or "sticky"

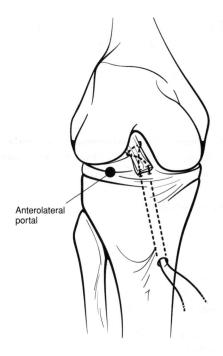

Anterolateral
portal

KNEE

COMPLICATIONS

- non-union or malunion of fragment
- incompetent ligament secondary to attenuation at time of injury prior to fracture
- infection

SELECTED REFERENCES

Hallam PJ, Fazal MA, Ashwood N, Ware HE, Glasgow MM, Powell JM. An alternative to fixation of displaced fractures of the anterior intercondylar eminence in children. J Bone Joint Surg Br 2002;84:579–582.

Osti L, Merlo F, Liu SH, Bocchi L. A simple modified arthroscopic procedure for fixation of displaced tibial eminence fractures. Arthroscopy 2000;16:379–382.

NOTES

_____
_____
_____
_____
_____
_____
_____

ARTHROSCOPICALLY AIDED TREATMENT OF INTERCONDYLAR SPINE AND/OR TUBEROSITY FRACTURE OF KNEE WITH FIXATION

CPT code   29851 arthroscopically aided treatment of intercondylar spine(s) and/or tuberosity fracture(s) of the knee, with or without manipulation; with internal or external fixation (includes arthroscopy)

ICD-9 code   823.00 fracture, tibial eminence

INDICATIONS

- tibial avulsion fractures rendering ACL or PCL incompetent with displacement of fragment

ALTERNATIVE TREATMENTS

- observation, casting in extension
- arthrotomy and repair
- same procedure without fixation (CPT code, 29850)

APPROACHES

Surgical Techniques

- standard knee arthroscopy with intra-articular manipulation of bone fragment into fracture base
- fixation done with screws or wires, if fragment large enough, or sutures through ligament and around bone fragment, if fragment is small, secured through tibial bone tunnel
- large fragment: temporary fixation with κ-wire and screw fixation
- small fragment: place sutures through or around fragment from anteromedial portal
- pass sutures through two drill holes made from anteromedial tibia into base of fracture/spine
- tie sutures over bone

POSTOPERATIVE MANAGEMENT

- crutches, non-weight-bearing
- immobilize for 1 week
- pain medication as needed

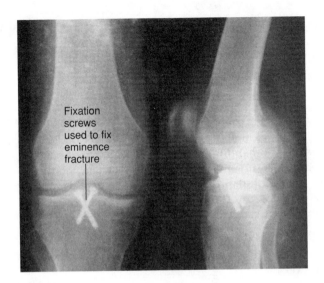

KNEE

REHABILITATION

- effusion reduction, straight leg raises, quadriceps activation with knee in extension
- begin active-assisted ROM postoperative week 1 and achieve full ROM, depending on fixation, by postoperative week 3
- partial weight bearing postoperative week 3 in brace
- active ROM, if fixation solid, postoperative week 3

COMPLICATIONS

- non-union or malunion of fragment
- instability due to interstitial ligament injury
- infection
- loss of extension

SELECTED REFERENCES

Reynders P, Reynders K, Broos P. Pediatric and adolescent tibial eminence fractures: arthroscopic cannulated screw fixation. J Trauma 2002;53:49–54.

Yip DK, Wong JW, Chien EP, Chan CF. Modified arthroscopic suture fixation of displaced tibial eminence fractures using a suture loop transporter. Arthroscopy 2001;17:101–106.

ARTHROSCOPICALLY AIDED TREATMENT OF TIBIAL FRACTURE, PROXIMAL (PLATEAU), BICONDYLAR

CPT code	29856 arthroscopically aided treatment of tibial fracture, proximal (plateau); bicondylar, with or without internal or external fixation (includes arthroscopy)
ICD-9 code	823.00 fracture, tibial plateau

INDICATION

- minimally displaced tibial plateau fracture

ALTERNATIVE TREATMENTS

- observation, casting in extension
- open arthrotomy with reduction and fixation

APPROACHES

- standard knee arthroscopy with manipulation of fracture to recreate congruent articular surface

Incision

- anterolateral incision over proximal lateral tibia

Surgical Techniques

- create bone window or open fracture site in lateral metaphysis
- elevate depressed fragments as necessary using arthroscopic viewing to monitor reduction
- reduction also monitored by C-arm image
- metaphyseal bone grafting as necessary to support and maintain reduction
- fixation done with screw, wires, and plate to maintain reduction

POSTOPERATIVE MANAGEMENT

- crutches, non-weight-bearing
- pain medication as needed

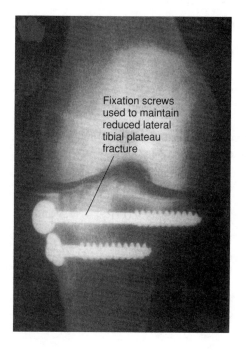

Fixation screws used to maintain reduced lateral tibial plateau fracture

REHABILITATION

- effusion reduction, straight leg raises, and quadriceps activation with knee in extension
- active ROM postoperative week 1
- non-weight-bearing for 6 weeks

COMPLICATIONS

- non-union or malunion
- failure to recreate smooth articular surface
- infection

SELECTED REFERENCES

Gill TJ, Moezzi DM, Oates KM, Sterett WI. Arthroscopic reduction and fixation of tibial plateau fractures in skiing. Clin Orthop 2001;383:243–249.

Kiefer H, Zivaljevic N, Imbriglia JE. Arthroscopic reduction and internal fixation of lateral tibial plateau fractures. Knee Surg Sports Traumatol Arthrosc 2001; 9:167–172.

ARTHROSCOPY, DIAGNOSTIC, WITH OR WITHOUT SYNOVIAL BIOPSY

CPT code   29870 arthroscopy, knee, diagnostic; with or without synovial biopsy
(separate procedure)

ICD-9 code   711.06 septic arthritis
714.0 rheumatoid arthritis
718.36 internal derangement

INDICATIONS

- unexplained knee pain or effusion and disability

ALTERNATIVE TREATMENTS

- observation
- arthrotomy

APPROACHES

- two or three portals
- lateral and medial parapatellar portals
- posteromedial and posterolateral portals as required
- superolateral or superomedial portal for outflow and/or patellofemoral tracking observation

Surgical Techniques

- systematic examination of entire intra-articular space
- valgus stress for medial compartment viewing and lateral gutter
- varus stress for lateral compartment viewing and medial gutter

POSTOPERATIVE MANAGEMENT

- crutches, weight bearing as tolerated
- pain medication as needed

REHABILITATION

- effusion reduction, straight leg raises, and quadriceps activation with knee in extension
- patellar mobilization
- advance activity as tolerated

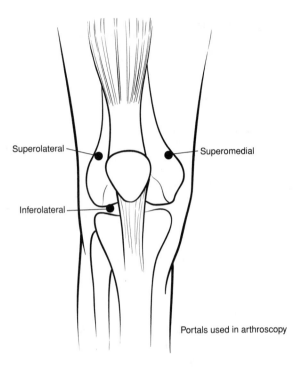

Portals used in arthroscopy

COMPLICATIONS

- stiffness and adhesions
- infection

SELECTED REFERENCES

Martinez A, Hechtman KS. Arthroscopic technique for the knee in morbidly obese patients. Arthroscopy 2002;18:E13.
Stetson WB, Templin K. Two- versus three-portal technique for routine knee arthroscopy. Am J Sports Med 2002;30:108–111.

NOTES

ARTHROSCOPY, KNEE, SURGICAL; FOR INFECTION, LAVAGE AND DRAINAGE

CPT code   29871 arthroscopy, knee, surgical; for infection, lavage and drainage

ICD-9 code   711.06 septic arthritis

INDICATIONS

- knee joint infection, any reason

ALTERNATIVE TREATMENTS

- serial aspirations
- open irrigation and drainage (arthrotomy)

APPROACHES

- two or three portals
  - anterior inferolateral and medial parapatellar portals
  - posteromedial and posterolateral portals as required for complete synovectomy and debridement of infected tissues

Surgical Techniques

- systematic examination of entire intra-articular space
- valgus stress for medial compartment viewing and lateral gutter
- varus stress for lateral compartment viewing and medial gutter
- debridement of all involved tissues, including grafts as appropriate and hardware if present
- leave drain for continued postoperative drainage and remove when drainage stops and/or postoperative day 2

POSTOPERATIVE MANAGEMENT

- crutches, weight bearing as tolerated
- pain medication as needed
- intravenous antibiotics, then orally for 6 weeks

REHABILITATION

- effusion reduction, straight leg raises, quadriceps activation with knee in extension
- patellar mobilization
- advance activity as tolerated

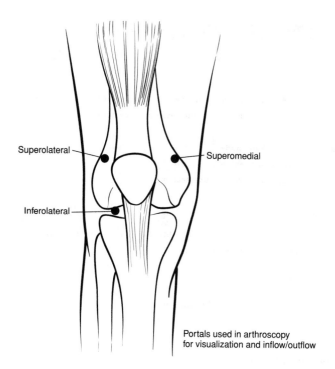

Portals used in arthroscopy
for visualization and inflow/outflow

COMPLICATIONS

- stiffness and adhesions
- continued infection

SELECTED REFERENCES

Ivey M, Clark R. Arthroscopic debridement of the knee for septic arthritis. Clin Orthop 1985;199:201–206.
Indelli PF, Dillingham M, Fanton G, Schurman DJ. Septic arthritis in postoperative anterior cruciate ligament reconstruction. Clin Orthop 2002;398:182–188.

NOTES

_____
_____
_____
_____
_____
_____
_____
_____

ARTHROSCOPY, KNEE, SURGICAL, REMOVAL OF LOOSE OR FOREIGN BODY

CPT code	29874 arthroscopy, knee, surgical; for removal of loose body or foreign body (e.g., osteochondritis dissecans fragmentation, chondral fragmentation)
ICD-9 code	717.60 loose body
	718.36 internal derangement
	732.7 osteochondritis dissecans

INDICATIONS

• intra-articular loose body causing pain, effusion, or mechanical symtoms
• bone, cartilage, foreign object

ALTERNATIVE TREATMENTS

• open irrigation and removal (arthrotomy)

APPROACHES

• two or three portals
    • locate loose body and diminish or stop in-flow of arthroscopic irrigant
    • use arthroscopic grasper to retieve
    • may have to use 18-gauge needle to impale loose body, to stabilize until it can be grasped with grasping instrument
    • may need to enlarge a portal for fragment removal
    • posteromedial and posterolateral portals as required to locate and remove all fragments

Surgical Techniques

• systematic examination of entire intra-articular space
• valgus stress for medial compartment viewing and lateral gutter
• varus stress for lateral compartment viewing and medial gutter

POSTOPERATIVE MANAGEMENT

• crutches, weight bearing as tolerated
• pain medication as needed
• intravenous antibiotics, then orally for 6 weeks

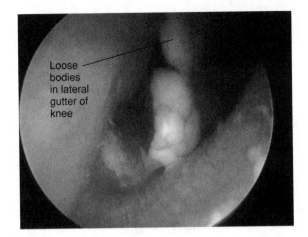

Loose bodies in lateral gutter of knee

REHABILITATION

- effusion reduction, straight leg raises, and quadriceps activation with knee in extension
- patellar mobilization
- advance activity as tolerated

COMPLICATIONS

- stiffness and adhesions
- infection
- arthritis

SELECTED REFERENCES

Aglietti P, Ciardullo A, Giron F, Ponteggia F. Results of arthroscopic excision of the fragment in the treatment of osteochondritis dissecans of the knee. Arthroscopy 2001;17:741–746.

Cain EL, Clancy WG. Treatment algorithm for osteochondral injuries of the knee. Clin Sports Med 2001;20:321–342.

NOTES

_____
_____
_____
_____
_____

ARTHROSCOPY, KNEE, SURGICAL, SYNOVECTOMY, LIMITED

CPT code	29875 arthroscopy, knee, surgical; synovectomy, limited (e.g., plica or shelf resection) (separate procedure)
ICD-9 code	727.00 synovitis
	727.83 plica

INDICATIONS

- recurrent effusion and/or pain from capsular fold
- mechanical symptoms: catching, locking
- failed conservative measures

ALTERNATIVE TREATMENTS

- injection with corticosteroid
- open irrigation and removal (arthrotomy)

APPROACHES

- standard knee arthroscopy, two or three portals

Surgical Techniques

- systematic examination of entire intra-articular space
- removal of inflamed or irritated synovial/capsular tissue where evidence of condylar scuffing seen
- plica typically observed as thickened, synovial fold draping over edge of medial femoral condyle and medial-to-medial facet of patella
- use mechanical shaver, electrocautery, or radiofrequency ablative device to resect plica

POSTOPERATIVE MANAGEMENT

- crutches, weight bearing as tolerated
- pain medication as needed

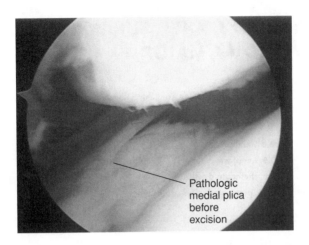

Pathologic
medial plica
before
excision

KNEE

REHABILITATION

- effusion reduction, straight leg raises, and quadriceps activation with knee in extension
- patellar mobilization
- advance activity as tolerated

COMPLICATIONS

- stiffness and adhesions
- infection
- hemarthrosis

SELECTED REFERENCES

Johnson DP, Eastwood DM, Witherow PJ. Symptomatic synovial plicae of the knee. J Bone Joint Surg Am 1993;75:1485–1496.
Ewing JW. Plica: pathologic or not? J Am Acad orthop Surg 1993;1:117–121.

NOTES

_____
_____
_____
_____
_____

ARTHROSCOPY, KNEE, SURGICAL, SYNOVECTOMY, MAJOR

CPT code	29876 arthroscopy, knee, surgical; synovectomy, major, two or more compartments (e.g., medial or lateral)
ICD-9 code	286.0 hemophilia
	213.9 neoplasm
	714.0 rheumatoid arthritis
	719.26 pigmented villonodular synovitis

INDICATIONS

- recurrent effusion and/or pain from synovitis
- failed conservative measures

ALTERNATIVE TREATMENTS

- injections, repeated aspiration
- open irrigation and removal (arthrotomy)
- radionuclide (P-32) synovectomy

APPROACHES

- standard knee arthroscopy, three or four portals
- begin in suprapatellar pouch and proceed with synovectomy using no. 4.5 and 5.5 synovial resector blade, electrocautery, or ablative device (radiofrequency)
- continue with medial compartment and lateral compartment debridement
- will require posteromedial and lateral portals for complete synovectomy

Surgical Techniques

- systematic review of entire intra-articular space
- removal of inflamed or irritated synovial/capsular tissue where evidence of condylar scuffing seen or with evidence of impingement within patellofemoral or tibiofemoral compartments

POSTOPERATIVE MANAGEMENT

- crutches, weight bearing as tolerated
- pain medication as needed

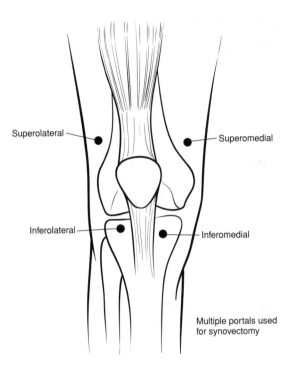

Superolateral

Superomedial

Inferolateral

Inferomedial

Multiple portals used
for synovectomy

REHABILITATION

- effusion reduction, straight leg raises, and quadriceps activation with knee in extension
- patellar mobilization
- advance activity as tolerated

COMPLICATIONS

- stiffness and adhesions
- infection, recurrent synovitis

SELECTED REFERENCES

Ogilvie-Harris DJ, Basinski A. Arthroscopic synovectomy of the knee for rheumatoid arthritis. Arthroscopy 1991;7:91–97.

Zvijac JE, Lau AC, Hechtman KS, Uribe JW, Tjin-A-Tsoi EW. Arthroscopic treatment of pigmented villonodular synovitis of the knee. Arthroscopy 1999; 15:613–617.

ARTHROSCOPY, KNEE, SURGICAL, DEBRIDEMENT AND SHAVING OF ARTICULAR CARTILAGE

CPT code   29877 arthroscopy, knee, surgical; debridement/shaving of articular cartilage (chondroplasty)

ICD-9 code   715.96 osteoarthritis

INDICATIONS

- failed conservative measures
- symptomatic click or pop or crepitation
- chondral lesion or fracture by examination and imaging studies

ALTERNATIVE TREATMENTS

- corticosteroid injections in older patients
- arthrotomy, removal and chondral sculpting

APPROACHES

- standard knee arthroscopy, two or three portals

Surgical Techniques

- systematic examination of entire intra-articular space
- chondral flap and or fragmentation removal
- debridement of articular surface to smooth stable edge with hand instruments or mechanical shaver (chondral biopsy as appropriate for possible future chondrocyte implantation)

POSTOPERATIVE MANAGEMENT

- crutches, weight bearing as tolerated
- pain medication as needed

REHABILITATION

- effusion reduction, straight leg raises, and quadriceps activation with knee in extension
- patellar mobilization
- advance activity as tolerated

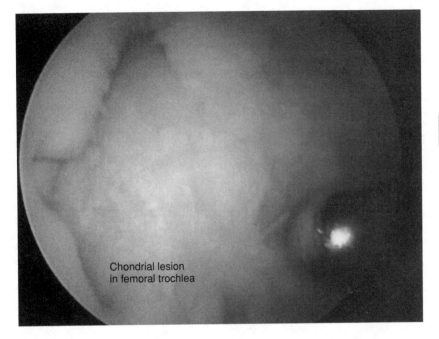

Chondrial lesion
in femoral trochlea

KNEE

COMPLICATIONS

- stiffness and adhesions
- infection

SELECTED REFERENCES

Dandy DJ. Arthroscopic debridement of the knee for osteoarthritis. J Bone Joint Surg Br 1991;73:877–878.
Wai EK, Kreder HJ, Williams JI. Arthroscopic debridement of the knee for osteoarthritis in patients fifty years or older: utilization and outcomes in the Province of Ontario. J Bone Joint Surg Am 2002;84-A:17–22.
Bert JM, Maschka K. The arthroscopic treatment of unicompartmental gonarthrosis: a five-year follow-up study of abrasion arthroplasty plus arthroscopic debridement and debridement alone. Arthroscopy 1989;5:25–32.

NOTES

_____
_____
_____
_____
_____
_____
_____

ARTHROSCOPY, KNEE, SURGICAL, ABRASION ARTHROPLASTY

CPT code   29879 arthroscopy, knee, surgical; abrasion arthroplasty (includes
                  chondroplasty where necessary) or multiple drilling or microfracture

ICD-9 code   715.96 osteoarthritis

INDICATIONS

- failed conservative measures
- chondral lesion on examination and confirmed by imaging studies

ALTERNATIVE TREATMENTS

- activity modification, wedges, NSAIDs
- unloader brace
- arthrotomy, removal and chondral sculpting

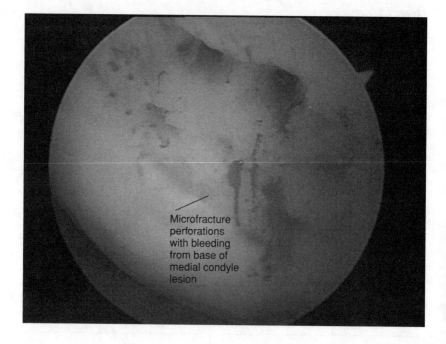

Microfracture
perforations
with bleeding
from base of
medial condyle
lesion

APPROACHES

- standard knee arthroscopy, two or three portals

Surgical Techniques

- systematic examination of entire intra-articular space
- debridement of articular surface to smooth stable edge
- microfracture with angled picks or drilling (with 0.625 mm pin) of exposed subchondral bone at 5-mm intervals
- ensure blood egress from sites with decrease in pump pressure and/or release of tourniquet
- (chondral biopsy for possible chondrocyte implantation in future)

KNEE

POSTOPERATIVE MANAGEMENT

- crutches, touch-down weight bearing for 6–8 weeks, continuous passive motion
- pain medication as needed

REHABILITATION

- effusion reduction, straight leg raises, quadriceps activation with knee in extension
- patellar mobilization
- minimal weight bearing to allow maturation of fibrocartilage (4 weeks optimal)

COMPLICATIONS

- stiffness and adhesions
- infection
- continued pain

SELECTED REFERENCES

Cain EL, Clancy WG. Treatment algorithm for osteochondral injuries of the knee. Clin Sports Med 2001;20:321–342.
Steadman JR, Rodkey WG, Rodrigo JJ. Microfracture: surgical technique and rehabilitation to treat chondral defects. Clin Orthop 2001;(391 Suppl):S362–369.

NOTES

_____

_____

_____

_____

_____

ARTHROSCOPY, KNEE, SURGICAL, WITH MENISCECTOMY (MEDIAL AND LATERAL)

CPT code　　　29880　arthroscopy, knee, surgical; with meniscectomy (medial and lateral, including any meniscal shaving)

ICD-9 codes　　836.0　torn medial meniscus
　　　　　　　　　836.1　torn lateral meniscus

INDICATIONS

- medial or lateral joint-line pain, tenderness, effusion, or mechanical symptoms not responding to conservative treatment

ALTERNATIVE TREATMENTS

- injections
- shoe wedges/orthotics, unloader bracing
- open meniscectomy

APPROACHES

- standard knee arthroscopy, two or three portals
- scope portal typically opposite compartment with meniscus tear; instruments through portal on same side as tear

Surgical Techniques

- systematic examination of entire intra-articular space
- partial meniscus excision as necessary to achieve stable rim, utilizing arthroscopic biters and shavers as appropriate
- preserve as much meniscal tissue as possible
- concurrent debridement of articular surface irregularities, synovitis, or pathologic plica problems as necessary

POSTOPERATIVE MANAGEMENT

- crutches, progress to full weight-bearing as tolerated
- pain medication as needed

REHABILITATION

- effusion reduction, straight leg raises, quadriceps activation with knee in extension
- patellar mobilization
- resume sports after effusion subsides, 3–6 weeks

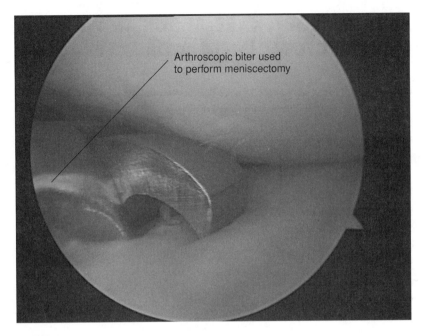

Arthroscopic biter used
to perform meniscectomy

COMPLICATIONS

- prolonged quadriceps atrophy
- post-meniscectomy arthritis
- infection

SELECTED REFERENCES

Hulet CH, Locker BG, Schiltz D, Texier A, Tallier E, Vielpeau CH. Arthroscopic
    medial meniscectomy on stable knees. J Bone Joint Surg Br 2001;83:29–32.
Juareguito JW, Elliot JS, Lietner T, Dixon LB, Reider B. The effects of arthroscopic
    partial lateral meniscectomy in an otherwise normal knee: a retrospective review
    of functional, clinical, and radiographic results. Arthroscopy 1995;11:29–36.

NOTES

ARTHROSCOPY, KNEE, SURGICAL, WITH MENISCECTOMY (MEDIAL OR LATERAL)

CPT code   29881 arthroscopy, knee, surgical; with menisectomy (medial or lateral, including any meniscal shaving)

ICD-9 codes   836.0 torn medial meniscus
                   836.1 torn lateral meniscus

INDICATIONS

- persistent joint-line pain, effusion, mechanical symptoms
- torn menisci, unrepairable

ALTERNATIVE TREATMENTS

- injections
- shoe wedges/orthotics, unloader bracing
- open meniscectomy

APPROACHES

- standard knee arthroscopy, two or three portals

Surgical Techniques

- systematic examination of entire intra-articular space
- partial meniscus excision as necessary to achieve stable rim, utilizing arthroscopic biters and shavers as appropriate
- concurrent debridement of articular surface irregularities, synovitis, and pathologic plica problems as necessary

POSTOPERATIVE MANAGEMENT

- pain medication as needed
- crutches as needed, progressive weight bearing

REHABILITATION

- effusion reduction, straight leg raises, and quadriceps activation with knee in extension
- patellar mobilization
- resume sports after effusion subsides, 3–6 weeks

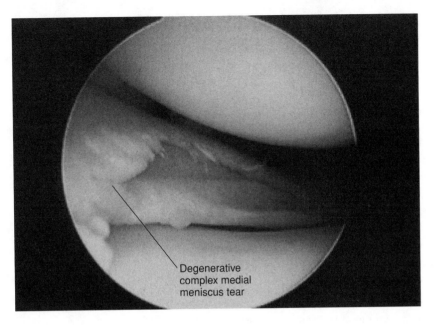

Degenerative
complex medial
meniscus tear

COMPLICATIONS

- prolonged quadriceps atrophy
- stiffness and adhesions
- infection
- post-meniscectomy arthritis

SELECTED REFERENCES

Chatain F, Robinson AH, Adeleine P, Chambat P, Neyret P. The natural history of the knee following arthroscopic medial meniscectomy. Knee Surg Sports Traumatol Arthrosc 2001;9:15–18.
Schimmer RC, Brulhart KB, Duff C, Glinz W. Arthroscopic partial meniscectomy: a 12-year follow-up and two-step evaluation of the long-term course. Arthroscopy 1998;14:136–142.

NOTES

ARTHROSCOPY, KNEE, SURGICAL, WITH MENISCUS REPAIR (MEDIAL TECHNIQUE)

CPT code   29882 arthroscopy, knee, surgical; with meniscus repair (medial or lateral)

ICD-9 code   836.0 torn medial meniscus

                    836.1 torn lateral meniscus

INDICATIONS

- torn medial-lateral meniscus within 3–4 mm of vascular supply and potential for healing after repair
- often occurs with anterior cruciate ligament injury

ALTERNATIVE TREATMENTS

- open meniscus repair
- activity modification, injections

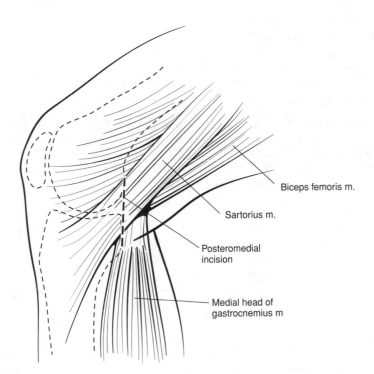

Biceps femoris m.

Sartorius m.

Posteromedial incision

Medial head of gastrocnemius m

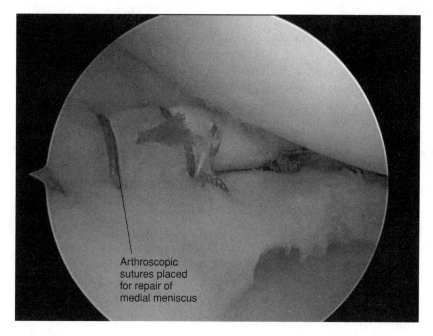

KNEE

Arthroscopic
sutures placed
for repair of
medial meniscus

APPROACHES

- standard knee arthroscopy, two or three portals

Incision

- posterolateral or posteromedial incisions for suture retrieval

Surgical Techniques—Medial Meniscus Technique

- posteromedial—incision 3 cm (1 cm above the joint line), slightly posterior to medial epicondyle, split sartorius fascia in-line with fibers, retract pes tendons posteriorly, create separation between medial gastrocnemius tendon and capsule (some tendons may need to be cut)
- sutures through cannula placed across tear and tied sequentially against posterior capsule
- alternative: absorbable fixation devices for repair

POSTOPERATIVE MANAGEMENT

- pain medication as needed
- crutches as needed

REHABILITATION

- effusion reduction, straight leg raises, and quadriceps activation with knee in extension
- patellar mobilization
- minimal weight-bearing for 6 weeks
- careful avoidance of axial compression with knee flexed more than 90°

COMPLICATIONS

- stiffness and adhesions
- infection
- failure of repair (10–25%)

SELECTED REFERENCES

Scott GA, Jolly BL, Henning CE. Combined posterior incision and arthroscopic intra-articular repair of the meniscus. An examination of factors affecting healing. J Bone Joint Surg Am 1986;68:847–861.

Rubman MH, Noyes FR, Barber-Westin SD. Arthroscopic repair of meniscal tears that extend into the avascular zone. A review of 198 single and complex tears. Am J Sports Med 1998;26:87–95.

NOTES

KNEE

ARTHROSCOPY, KNEE, SURGICAL, WITH MENISCUS REPAIR (LATERAL TECHNIQUE)

CPT code   29882 arthroscopy, knee, surgical; with meniscus repair (medial or lateral)

ICD-9 code   836.0 torn medial meniscus

                    836.1 torn lateral meniscus

INDICATIONS

- torn medial-lateral meniscus within 3–4 mm of vascular supply and potential for healing after repair
- often occurs with anterior cruciate ligament injury

ALTERNATIVE TREATMENTS

- open meniscus repair
- activity modification, injections

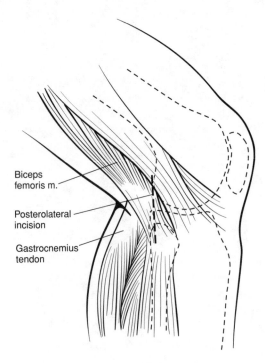

Biceps femoris m.

Posterolateral incision

Gastrocnemius tendon

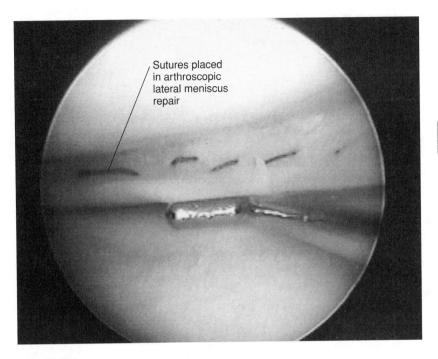

Sutures placed
in arthroscopic
lateral meniscus
repair

APPROACHES

- standard knee arthroscopy, two or three portals

Incision

- posterolateral or posteromedial incisions for suture retrieval

Surgical Techniques—Lateral Meniscus Technique

- posterolateral—incision 3 cm (1 cm above the joint line), slightly posterior to LCL; split iliotibial band in-line with fibers, and create separation between lateral gastrocnemius tendon and capsule
- sutures through cannula placed across tear and tied sequentially against posterior capsule
- alternative: absorbable fixation devices for repair

POSTOPERATIVE MANAGEMENT

- pain medication as needed
- crutches as needed

REHABILITATION

- effusion reduction, straight leg raises, and quadriceps activation with knee in extension
- patellar mobilization
- minimal weight-bearing for 6 weeks
- careful avoidance of axial compression with knee flexed more than 90°

COMPLICATIONS

- stiffness and adhesions
- infection; neurovascular injury: popliteal artery, saphenous nerve, peroneal nerve
- failure of repair (10–25%)

SELECTED REFERENCES

Scott GA, Jolly BL, Henning CE. Combined posterior incision and arthroscopic intra-articular repair of the meniscus. An examination of factors affecting healing. J Bone Joint Surg Am 1986;68:847–861.

Rubman MH, Noyes FR, Barber-Westin SD. Arthroscopic repair of meniscal tears that extend into the avascular zone. A review of 198 single and complex tears. Am J Sports Med 1998;26:87–95.

KNEE

NOTES

_____

_____

_____

_____

_____

_____

_____

_____

ARTHROSCOPY, KNEE, SURGICAL, WITH LYSIS OF ADHESIONS

CPT code	29884 arthroscopy, knee, surgical; with lysis of adhesions, with or without manipulation (separate procedure)
ICD-9 code	718.46 contracture
	718.56 arthrofibrosis

INDICATIONS

- persistent pain within joint with or without restricted motion
- anterior nodule post reconstruction ACL
- peripatellar adhesions, fibrosis after total knee arthroplasty

ALTERNATIVE TREATMENTS

- manipulation under anesthesia
- activity modification, injections

APPROACHES

- standard knee arthroscopy, two or three portals
- posterolateral or posteromedial portals for improved access to joint for complete lysis
- systematic review of entire intra-articular space

Surgical Techniques

- scar and adhesion resection with shaver, arthroscopic biter, and/or electrocautery
- resection of medial and lateral peripatellar adhesions
- may require release of adhesions between inferopatellar tendon and proximal, anterior tibia
- resection should include all areas of joint, with care to achieve normal motion and normal patellar mobility (lateral and sometimes medial capsular release may be necessary)
- care should be taken to achieve hemostasis
- consider steroid injection at end of procedure to limit postoperative scar formation

POSTOPERATIVE MANAGEMENT

- pain medication as needed
- crutches as needed
- consider continuous passive motion at home or in hospital, continuous epidural if in hospital as needed during first few days of mobilization

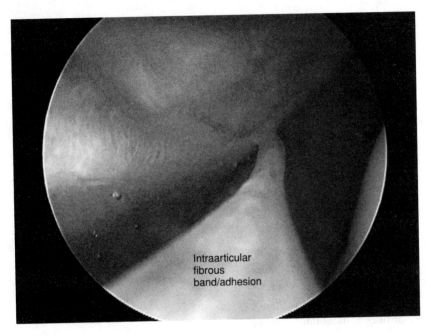

KNEE

Intraarticular
fibrous
band/adhesion

REHABILITATION

- effusion reduction, straight leg raises, and quadriceps activation with knee in extension
- patellar mobilization
- dynamic extension bracing
- minimal weight-bearing for 6 weeks

COMPLICATIONS

- stiffness and adhesions
- infection
- recurrent loss of motion, pain

SELECTED REFERENCES

Cosgarea AJ, DeHaven KE, Lovelock JE. The surgical treatment of arthrofibrosis of the knee. Am J Sports Med 1994;22:184–191.
Shelbourne KD, Patel DV, Martini DJ. Classification and management of arthrofibrosis of the knee after anterior cruciate ligament reconstruction. Am J Sports Med 1996;24:857–862.

ARTHROSCOPY, KNEE, SURGICAL, DRILLING FOR OSTEOCHONDRITIS DISSECANS WITH BONE GRAFTING

CPT code   29885 arthroscopy, knee, surgical; drilling for osteochondritis dissecans (OCD) with bone grafting, with or without internal fixation (including debridement of base of lesion)

ICD-9 code   732.7 osteochondritis dissecans, knee

INDICATIONS

- osteochondritis dissecans of femoral condyles, lesion loose but still attached with osseous component

ALTERNATIVE TREATMENTS

- observation with or without casting
- drilling without bone grafting

APPROACHES

- standard knee arthroscopy, two or three portals
- small arthrotomy for access to lesion and placement of bone graft (may be accomplished arthroscopically if direct access possible through scope portals)

Incision

- small incision over bone-graft harvest site (Gerdy's tubercle in field or iliac crest), cancellous bone preferred

Surgical Techniques

- systematic review of entire intra-articular space
- define extent of lesion and ensure congruency of fit
- "lift" fragment and place bone graft in base
- replace lesion and "compress" to allow articular congruency
- fix lesion with headless screws or bioabsorbable pins to stabilize

POSTOPERATIVE MANAGEMENT

- pain medication as needed
- crutches until healed

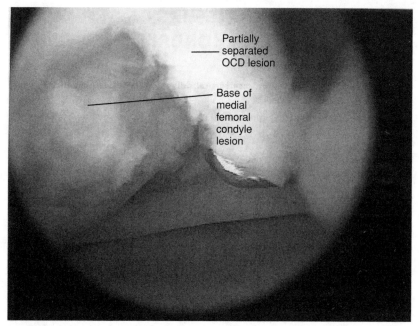

Partially separated OCD lesion

Base of medial femoral condyle lesion

KNEE

REHABILITATION

- effusion reduction, straight leg raises, and quadriceps activation with knee in extension
- patellar mobilization
- minimal weight bearing for 6 weeks

COMPLICATIONS

- infection
- loss of fixation or avascular necrosis of fragment
- failure of healing

SELECTED REFERENCES

Victoroff BN, Marcus RE, Deutsch A. Arthroscopic bone peg fixation in the treatment of osteochondritis dissecans of the knee. Arthroscopy 1996;12:506–509.
Johnson LL, Uitvlugt G, Austin MD, Detrisac DA, Johnson C. Osteochondritis dissecans of the knee: arthroscopic compression screw fixation. Arthroscopy 1990;6:179–189.

ARTHROSCOPY, KNEE, SURGICAL, DRILLING FOR INTACT OSTEOCHONDRITIS DISSECANS

CPT code   29886 arthroscopy, knee, surgical; drilling for intact osteochondritis dissecans

ICD-9 code   732.7 osteochondritis dissecans, knee

INDICATIONS

- osteochondritis dissecans of femoral condyles, lesion in place without evidence of subchondral bone or articular surface fissuring

ALTERNATIVE TREATMENTS

- observation with or without casting
- drilling with fixation

APPROACHES

- standard knee arthroscopy, two or three portals
- retrograde drilling device (ACL tibial tunnel guide or equivalent, i.e., Microvector)
- use small, smooth K-wire and make multiple perforations

Surgical Techniques

- systematic review of entire intra-articular space
- define extent of lesion and assure congruency of fit
- drill antegrade through subchondral bone without penetrating the chondral surface
- retrograde drilling using 1.6– or 2.0–mm K-wire if unable to accurately drill in retrograde fashion

POSTOPERATIVE MANAGEMENT

- pain medication as needed
- crutches until healed

REHABILITATION

- effusion reduction, straight leg raises, and quadriceps activation with knee in extension
- patellar mobilization
- minimal weight-bearing for 6 weeks

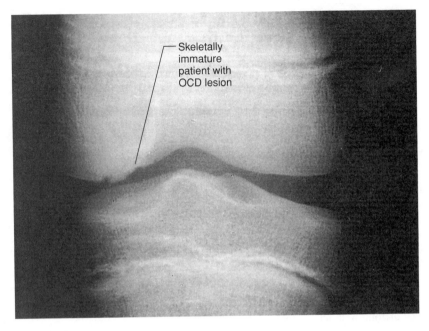

Skeletally immature patient with OCD lesion

COMPLICATIONS

- infection
- persistent non-union
- loss of fixation or avascular necrosis of fragment

SELECTED REFERENCES

Kocher MS, Micheli LJ, Yaniv M, Zurakowski D, Ames A, Adrignolo AA. Functional and radiographic outcome of juvenile osteochondritis dissecans of the knee treated with transarticular arthroscopic drilling. Am J Sports Med 2001;29:562–566.
Aglietti P, Buzzi R, Bassi PB, Fioriti M. Arthroscopic drilling in juvenile osteochondritis dissecans of the medial femoral condyle. Arthroscopy 1994;10:286–291.

NOTES

ARTHROSCOPY, KNEE, SURGICAL, DRILLING FOR INTACT OSTEOCHONDRITIS DISSECANS WITH INTERNAL FIXATION

CPT code   **29887** arthroscopy, knee, surgical; drilling for intact osteochondritis dissecans
with internal fixation

ICD-9 code   **732.7** osteochondritis dissecans, knee

INDICATIONS

- pain, effusion, compromise of function
- osteochondritis dissecans of femoral condyles, lesion in place without evidence of subchondral bone or articular surface fissuring

ALTERNATIVE TREATMENTS

- observation with or without casting
- drilling without fixation

APPROACHES

- standard knee arthroscopy, two or three portals
- retrograde drilling device (ACL tibial tunnel guide or equivalent, i.e., Microvector)
- accessory portals as possible to allow direct access to lesion

SURGICAL TECHNIQUE

- systematic review of entire intra-articular space
- define extent of lesion and ensure congruency of fit
- antegrade drilling to reduce articular surface penetration
- retrograde drilling if unable to accurately drill in antegrade fashion
- fixation perpendicular to articular and lesion surfaces using headless screws or bioabsorbable pins

POSTOPERATIVE MANAGEMENT

- pain medication as needed
- crutches until healed

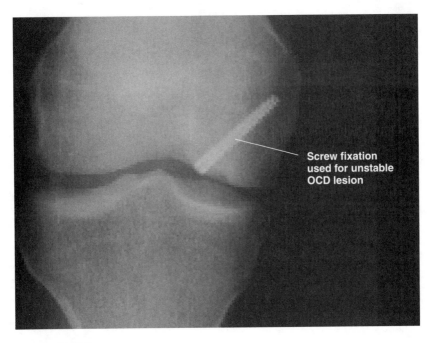

Screw fixation
used for unstable
OCD lesion

KNEE

REHABILITATION

- effusion reduction, straight leg raises, and quadriceps activation with knee in extension
- patellar mobilization
- minimal weight-bearing for 6 weeks

COMPLICATIONS

- infection
- loss of fixation or avascular necrosis of fragment
- failure to obtain bone healing

SELECTED REFERENCES

Cugat R, Garcia M, Cusco X, Monllau JC, Vilaro J, Juan X, Ruiz-Cotorro A. Osteochondritis dissecans: a historical review and it treatment with cannulated screws. Arthroscopy 1993;9:675–684.

Friedrerichs MG, Greis PE, Burks RT. Pitfalls associated with fixation of osteochondritis dissecans fragments using bioabsorbable screws. Arthroscopy 2001;17:542–545.

ARTHROSCOPICALLY AIDED ANTERIOR CRUCIATE LIGAMENT REPAIR, ALLOGRAFT

CPT code   **29888** arthroscopically aided anterior cruciate ligament repair/augmentation or reconstruction (allograft)

ICD-9 code   **844.2** torn anterior cruciate ligament

INDICATIONS

- ACL rupture with instability
- revision ACL reconstruction
- multiple ligament reconstruction

ALTERNATIVE TREATMENTS

- observation with bracing
- extra-articular ACL reconstruction

APPROACHES

- standard knee arthroscopy, two or three portals

Incision

- small incision over anteromedial tibia for drilling of tibial tunnel

Surgical Techniques

- prepare allograft and pre-tension to remove crimp
- drill tibial tunnel through ACL footprint (slightly medial to midline)
- dilate or drill tunnel to appropriate diameter for prepared graft
- locate femoral tunnel location and drill to depth as per protocol of fixation device (minimum of 20 mm) (femoral tunnel should be at 1:30 position in a left knee, as far posterior as possible without breaking posterior cortex)
- pass graft and fix with fixation device in femoral tunnel
- cycle knee to remove crimp
- fix tibial end of graft with appropriate graft tension, posterior drawer applied, and knee in approximately 20° of knee flexion
- allograft bone–patellar tendon–bone

POSTOPERATIVE MANAGEMENT

- pain medication as needed
- crutches until limp eliminated

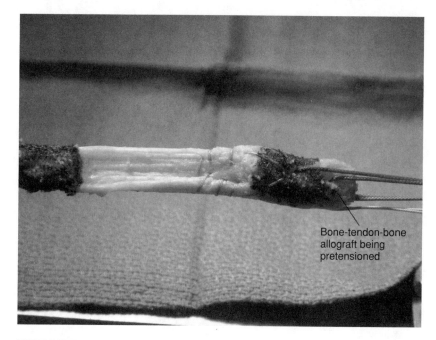

Bone-tendon-bone allograft being pretensioned

REHABILITATION

- effusion reduction, straight leg raises, quadriceps activation, and patellar mobilization
- progressive exercises as per protocol

COMPLICATIONS

- infection, disease transmission
- failure of integration/ligamentization; loss of extension
- re-rupture (10%) or recurrent instability

SELECTED REFERENCES

Noyes FR, Barber-Westin SD. Allograft reconstruction of the anterior and posterior cruciate ligaments: report of ten-year experience and results. Instr Course Lect 1993;42:381–396.

Noyes FR, Barber-Westin SD. Revision anterior cruciate ligament reconstruction: report of 11–year experience and results in 114 consecutive patients. Instr Course Lect 2001;50:451–461.

ARTHROSCOPICALLY AIDED ANTERIOR CRUCIATE LIGAMENT REPAIR, BONE–PATELLAR TENDON–BONE GRAFT

CPT code   **29888** arthroscopically aided anterior cruciate ligament repair/augmentation or reconstruction (bone–patellar tendon–bone graft)

ICD-9 code   **844.2** torn anterior cruciate ligament

INDICATIONS

- ACL rupture with symptomatic buckling or giving way

ALTERNATIVE TREATMENTS

- observation with bracing
- extra-articular ACL reconstruction

APPROACHES

- standard knee arthroscopy, two or three portals
- small incision for harvesting of graft over patellar tendon, harvesting of central third with bone plugs from patella and tibial tubercle, do not "isolate" tendon at medial and lateral borders to avoid devascularizing remaining tendon

Surgical Techniques

- repair and/or excise meniscal lesions as appropriate
- drill tibial tunnel through ACL footprint (slightly medial to midline and avoiding anterior impingement)
- dilate or drill tunnel to appropriate diameter for prepared graft
- locate femoral tunnel location and drill to depth to accommodate bone plug (femoral tunnel should be at 1:30 position in a left knee, as far posterior as possible without breaking posterior cortex)
- pass graft and fix with interference screw in femoral tunnel
- cycle knee to remove crimp
- fix tibial end of graft with appropriate graft tension, posterior drawer applied and knee in 0°–20° of knee flexion
- close paratenon over harvest, bone graft, patella, and tibial tubercle if possible

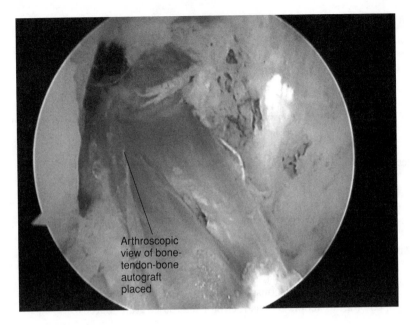

Arthroscopic
view of bone-
tendon-bone
autograft
placed

KNEE

POSTOPERATIVE MANAGEMENT

- pain medication as needed
- crutches until limp eliminated

REHABILITATION

- effusion reduction, straight leg raises, quadriceps activation, and patellar mobilization
- progressive exercises as per protocol

COMPLICATIONS

- infection; patellar fracture; patellar tendon rupture
- loss of extension
- re-rupture (10%) or recurrent instability

SELECTED REFERENCES

Bach BR, Levy ME, Bojchuk J, Tradonsky S, Bush-Joseph CA, Khan NH. Single incision endoscopic anterior cruciate ligament reconstruction using patellar tendon autograft. Minimum two-year follow-up evaluation. Am J Sports Med 1998;26:30–40.

Plancher KD, Steadman JR, Briggs KK, Hutton KS. Reconstruction of the anterior cruciate ligament in patients who are at least forty years old. A long-term follow-up and outcome study. J Bone Joint Surg Am 1998;80:184–197.

ARTHROSCOPICALLY AIDED ANTERIOR CRUCIATE LIGAMENT REPAIR, HAMSTRING GRAFT

CPT code   **29888** arthroscopically aided anterior cruciate ligament repair/augmentation or reconstruction (hamstring graft)

ICD-9 code   **844.2** torn anterior cruciate ligament

INDICATIONS

- ACL rupture with symptomatic buckling or giving way

ALTERNATIVE TREATMENTS

- Observation with bracing
- extra-articular ACL reconstruction
- open or arthroscopic reconstruction using other graft source

APPROACHES

- standard knee arthroscopy, two or three portals

Incision

- small incision for harvesting of graft over tibial insertion of pes tendons

Surgical Techniques

- use tendon stripper to harvest tendon after freeing from all fascial attachments
- debride stump and perform limited notchplasty
- drill tibial tunnel through ACL footprint (slightly medial to midline and at border of inner edge of lateral meniscus anterior horn)
- dilate or drill tunnel to appropriate diameter for prepared graft
- locate femoral tunnel location and drill to depth as per protocol of fixation device (minimum of 20 mm) (femoral tunnel should be at 1:30 position in a left knee, as far posterior as possible without breaking posterior cortex)
- pass graft and fix with chosen fixation device in femoral tunnel
- cycle knee to remove crimp
- fix tibial end of graft with appropriate graft tension, posterior drawer applied, and knee in approximately 20° of knee flexion

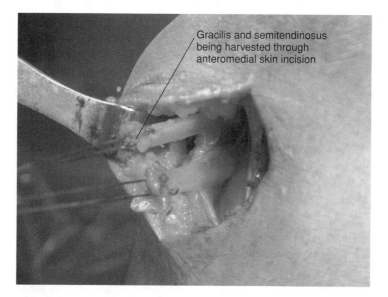

Gracilis and semitendinosus being harvested through anteromedial skin incision

POSTOPERATIVE MANAGEMENT

- pain medication as needed
- crutches until limp eliminated

REHABILITATION

- effusion reduction, straight leg raises, quadriceps activation, and patellar mobilization
- protected weight-bearing for 3–4 weeks
- progressive exercises as per protocol

COMPLICATIONS

- loss of motion
- infection, hamstring weakness
- re-rupture (10%) or recurrent instability

SELECTED REFERENCES

Pinczewski LA, Deehan DJ, Salmon LJ, Russell VJ, Clingeleffer A. A five-year comparison of patellar tendon versus four-strand hamstring tendon autograft for arthroscopic reconstruction of the anterior cruciate ligament. Am J Sports Med 2002;30:523–536.

Shaib MD, Kan DM, Chang SK, Marumoto JM, Richardson AB. A prospective randomized comparison of patellar tendon versus semitendinosus and gracilis tendon autografts for anterior cruciate ligament reconstruction. Am J Sports Med 2002;30:214–220.

ARTHROSCOPICALLY AIDED POSTERIOR CRUCIATE LIGAMENT REPAIR, ALL ARTHROSCOPIC

CPT code   29889 arthroscopically aided posterior cruciate ligament repair/augmentation
or reconstruction (all arthroscopic procedure)

ICD-9 code   844.8 torn posterior cruciate ligament

INDICATIONS

- PCL rupture with symptomatic buckling or giving way, or progressive patellofemoral arthrosis and symptoms
- multiple knee ligament injury

ALTERNATIVE TREATMENTS

- observation with bracing
- extra-articular PCL reconstruction

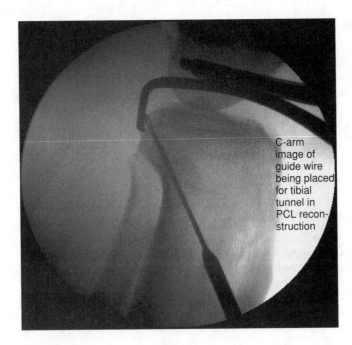

C-arm image of guide wire being placed for tibial tunnel in PCL reconstruction

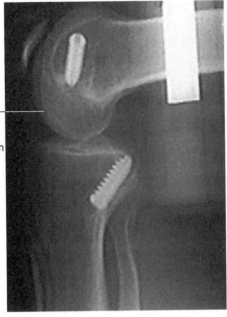

Postoperative radiograph with fixation screws for PCL restoration

KNEE

APPROACHES

- standard knee arthroscopy, two or three portals
- utilize posterior-medial portal to debride PCL stump, tibial attachment
- prepare tibial tunnel
- graft passage

Surgical Techniques

- harvest and prepare autograft or allograft
- incision as necessary to expose anteromedial tibia for tibial tunnel drilling; use C-arm and protect guide wire from popliteal artery
- guide wire should exit posterior tibia 12–17 mm below joint
- drill 11–13 mm tunnel
- femoral tunnel prepared over guide wire placed from medial epicondylar area to 11 o'clock for left knee (1 o'clock for right) and 8–10 mm proximal to articular edge (alternate method: drill from inferolateral portal into femoral origin and exit medially)
- pass graft(s) and cycle knee to remove crimp
- fix graft with knee at 90° flexion and anterior drawer applied recreating tibial step-off

POSTOPERATIVE MANAGEMENT

- pain medication as needed
- immobilization in extension, progressive weight bearing for 3–4 weeks

REHABILITATION

- effusion reduction, straight leg raises, quadriceps activation, and patellar mobilization
- progressive ROM, strengthening of quadriceps
- return to sports at 9 months

COMPLICATIONS

- re-rupture or recurrent instability
- infection
- loss of flexion

SELECTED REFERENCES

Fanelli GC, Giannotti BF, Edson CJ. Arthroscopically assisted combined anterior and posterior cruciate ligament reconstruction. Arthroscopy 1996;12:5–14.
Clancy WG. Repair and reconstruction of the posterior cruciate ligament. In: Chapman MW, ed. Operative orthopaedics, 2nd ed. Philadelphia: Lippincott, 1993:2093–2107.

NOTES

KNEE

ARTHROSCOPICALLY AIDED POSTERIOR CRUCIATE LIGAMENT REPAIR, TIBIAL INLAY PROCEDURE

CPT code	29889 arthroscopically aided posterior cruciate ligament repair/augmentation reconstruction (tibial inlay procedure)
ICD-9 code	844.8 torn posterior cruciate ligament

INDICATIONS

- PCL rupture with symptomatic buckling or giving way, or progressive patellofemoral arthrosis and symptoms

ALTERNATIVE TREATMENTS

- observation with bracing
- osteotomy

APPROACHES

- standard knee arthroscopy, two or three portals

Incision

- incision depends on graft used: bone–tendon–bone, hamstrings, or prepare allografts

Surgical Techniques

- prepare femoral tunnel from medial epicondyle to 11 o'clock for left knee (1 o'clock for right knee), 8–10 mm posterior to articular edge
- place suture passing device from femoral tunnel toward posterior capsule
- popliteal incision or inverted hockey stick incision along medial gastrocnemius and curve along popliteal flexion crease
- split interval between semimembranosus and medial gastrocnemius laterally for posterior tibial exposure and capsulotomy
- create tibial trough; drill 3.2-mm hole in bony end of graft; drill 3.2-mm hole in proximal tibia from posterior to anterior, and fix graft with 4.5- or 6.5-mm screw
- use suture-passing device to pass femoral portion of graft from posterior exposure into femoral tunnel
- cycle knee 20 times and fix femoral portion of graft with interference screw or ligament button

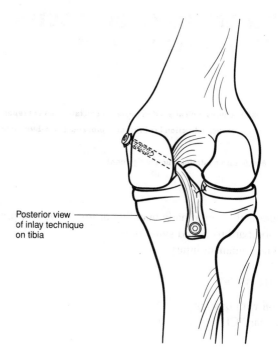

Posterior view
of inlay technique
on tibia

POSTOPERATIVE MANAGEMENT

- pain medication as needed
- crutches until limp eliminated

REHABILITATION

- immobilize knee at 0 degrees with partial weight-bearing for 3–4 weeks
- effusion reduction, straight leg raises, quadriceps activation rehabilitation, and patellar mobilization
- progressive exercises as per protocol

COMPLICATIONS

- re-rupture (10%) or recurrent instability
- infection, loss of motion

SELECTED REFERENCES

Berg EE. Posterior cruciate ligament tibial inlay reconstruction. Arthroscopy 1995;11:69–76.

Graham SM, Parker RD, McAllister DR, Calabrese GJ. Tibial inlay technique for posterior cruciate reconstruction. Tech Orthop 2001;16:136–147.

ARTHROSCOPICALLY AIDED POSTERIOR CRUCIATE LIGAMENT REPAIR, TWO-BUNDLE TECHNIQUE

CPT code   **29889** arthroscopically aided posterior cruciate ligament repair/augmentation or reconstruction (arthroscopic procedure two-bundle technique)

ICD-9 code   **844.8** torn posterior cruciate ligament

INDICATIONS

- PCL rupture with symptomatic buckling or giving way, or progressive patellofemoral arthrosis and symptoms
- multiple knee ligament injury

ALTERNATIVE TREATMENTS

- observation with bracing
- extra-articular PCL reconstruction

APPROACHES

- standard knee arthroscopy, two or three portals
- utilize posterior-medial portal to debride PCL stump, tibial attachment; prepare tibial tunnel; graft passage

Surgical Techniques

- harvest, prepare autograft or allograft
- incision as necessary to expose anteromedial tibia for tibial tunnel drilling; use C-arm and protect guide wire from popliteal artery
- guide wire should exit posterior tibia 12–17 mm below joint
- drill 11–13 mm tunnel
- femoral tunnel prepared over guide wire placed from medial epicondylar area to 11 o'clock for left knee (1 o'clock for right knee), 8–11 mm posterior to articular margin
- place second guide wire 12–15 mm posterior to first
- make anterolateral tunnel 8–9 mm in diameter
- make posteromedial tunnel 6–7 mm
- pass graft(s) and cycle knee to remove crimp
- fix anterolateral bundle graft with knee at 90° flexion and anterior drawer applied, recreating tibial step-off; fix posteromedial bundle at 30° flexion
- perform routine closure

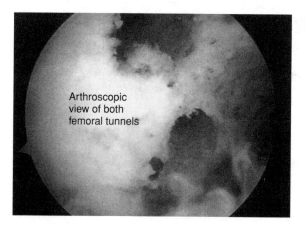

Arthroscopic view of both femoral tunnels

POSTOPERATIVE MANAGEMENT

- pain medication as needed
- immobilization in extension, restricted weight bearing for 3–4 weeks

REHABILITATION

- effusion reduction, straight leg raises, quadriceps activation, and patellar mobilization
- progressive ROM, strengthening of quadriceps
- return to sports at 9 months

COMPLICATIONS

- re-rupture or recurrent instability
- infection
- loss of flexion

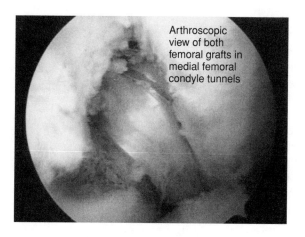

Arthroscopic view of both femoral grafts in medial femoral condyle tunnels

SELECTED REFERENCES

Trawick RH, Blair BA. Double-tunnel technique for the reconstruction of the posterior cruciate ligament. Tech Orthop 2001;16:127–135.

Harner C, Janaushek M, Kanamori A, et al. Biomechanical analysis of a double-bundle posterior cruciate ligament reconstruction. Am J Sports Med 2000;28:144–151.

NOTES

_____

_____

_____

_____

_____

_____

_____

_____

_____

_____

KNEE

PART IV

HIP, FOOT, & ANKLE

ARTHROSCOPY OF HIP, LOOSE BODY REMOVAL

CPT Code   **29861** arthroscopy of hip, loose body removal

ICD-9 Code   **718.15** loose body, hip
                  718.95 internal derangement

INDICATIONS

- mechanical locking, catching, popping with motion, not relieved with rest, rehabilitation, or NSAIDs
- pain relieved by intra-articular injection of anesthetic
- positive imaging study: radiographs, CT-arthrography, or MRI

ALTERNATIVE TREATMENT

- arthrotomy and removal

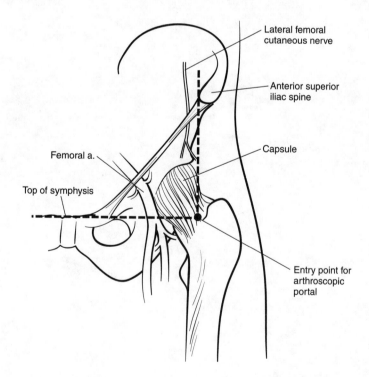

Lateral femoral cutaneous nerve

Anterior superior iliac spine

Capsule

Femoral a.

Top of symphysis

Entry point for arthroscopic portal

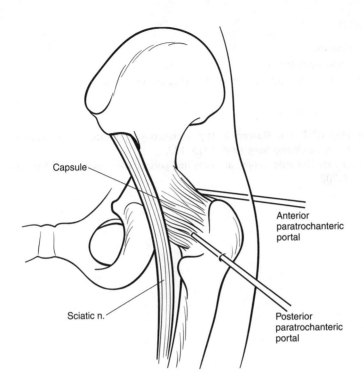

Capsule

Anterior
paratrochanteric
portal

HIP, FOOT,
& ANKLE

Sciatic n.

Posterior
paratrochanteric
portal

APPROACHES

- supine
- lateral decubitus

Surgical Techniques

- place limb in traction and distract
- vent the capsule with 18-gauge needle
- create lateral portal for initial viewing along superior margin of greater trochanter at anterior border
- create direct anterior portal by sagittal line from anterior-superior iliac spine (ASIS), intersecting transverse line from tip of greater trochanter
- inspect joint and use shaver and hand instruments to debride chondral lesions, loose bodies, synovium

POSTOPERATIVE MANAGEMENT

- crutches for comfort for 1–3 days, early motion
- active ROM, PREs, cycling

COMPLICATIONS

- infection
- wound hematoma
- neurovascular injury (femoral nerve, artery, vein)

SELECTED REFERENCES

McCarthy JC, Day B, Busconi B. Hip arthroscopy: applications and technique. J Am Acad Orthop Surg 1995;3:115–122.
Sweeney HJ Hip arthroscopy: anatomy and portals. Clin Sports Med 2001;20: 697–702.

NOTES

_____

_____

_____

_____

_____

_____

_____

_____

_____

_____

HIP, FOOT,
& ANKLE

ARTHROSCOPY OF HIP, DEBRIDEMENT OF LABRAL TEAR

CPT Code   **29862 arthroscopy of hip, debridement of labral tear**

ICD-9 Code   **718.15 loose body**
                   718.95 internal derangement

INDICATIONS

- mechanical locking, catching, popping with motion not relieved with rest, rehabilitation, or NSAIDs
- pain relieved by intra-articular injection of anesthetic
- positive imaging study: radiographs, CT-arthrography, or MRI

ALTERNATIVE TREATMENT

- arthrotomy and debridement

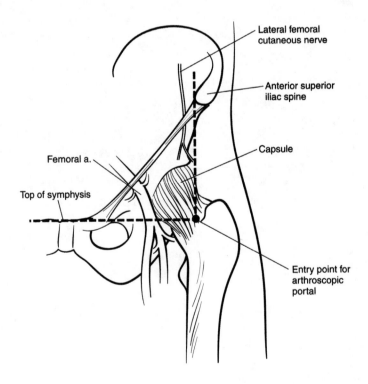

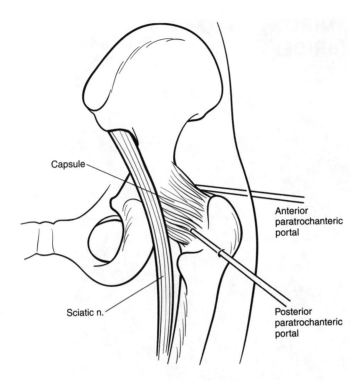

Capsule

Anterior
paratrochanteric
portal

Sciatic n.

Posterior
paratrochanteric
portal

APPROACHES

- supine
- lateral decubitus

Surgical Techniques

- place limb in traction and distract
- vent the capsule with 18-gauge needle
- create lateral portal for initial viewing along superior margin of greater trochanter at anterior border
- create direct anterior portal by sagittal line from ASIS, intersecting transverse line from tip of greater trochanter
- inspect joint and use shaver and hand instruments to debride torn labrum

POSTOPERATIVE MANAGEMENT

- crutches for comfort for 1–3 days, early motion
- active ROM, PREs, cycling

HIP, FOOT,
& ANKLE

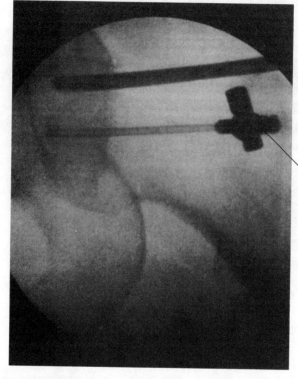

Radiographic
C-arm image
of arthroscope
and flow cannula

COMPLICATIONS

- infection
- wound hematoma
- neurovascular injury (femoral nerve, artery, vein)

SELECTED REFERENCES

Byrd JWT. Labral lesions: an elusive source of hip pain. Arthroscopy
  1996;12:603–612.
McCarthy JC, Day B, Busconi B. Hip arthroscopy: applications and technique.
  J Am Acad Orthop Surg 1995;3:115–122.

NOTES

_____

_____

_____

_____

_____

_____

_____

_____

_____

_____

HIP, FOOT,
& ANKLE

INCISION, DECOMPRESSION FASCIOTOMY, LEG

CPT code	27600	incision, decompression fasciotomy, leg; anterior and/or lateral compartments only
	27601	incision, posterior compartment(s) only
	27602	incision, anterior and/or lateral, and posterior compartments

ICD-9 code	958.8	exertional compartment syndrome of the leg

INDICATIONS

- leg pain associated with exercise, unrelieved with nonoperative measures, AND
- elevated compartment pressures
  - pre-exercise $\geq$ 15 mm Hg
  - 1 minute postexercise $\geq$ 30 mm Hg
  - 5 minutes postexercise $\geq$ 20 mm Hg

ALTERNATIVE TREATMENTS

- nonoperative—stretching, alternative activities
- activity modification to avoid painful exercise
- endoscopic fasciotomy

APPROACHES

Surgical Techniques
- anterior and/or lateral compartment—anterolateral longitudinal incision over distal one third of leg
  - identify and protect superficial peroneal nerve branches
  - incise fascia of compartment(s) proximally and distally with long Metzenbaum scissors
- posterior compartments
  - medial incision over mid-third of leg
  - identify and protect saphenous vein and nerve
  - incise fascia of superficial and deep compartments proximally and distally with long Metzenbaum scissors
  - may need to elevate flexor digitorum longus (FDL) from tibia to incise fascia of tibialis posterior muscle (fifth compartment)

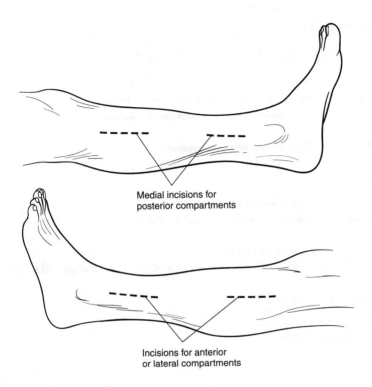

Medial incisions for
posterior compartments

Incisions for anterior
or lateral compartments

POSTOPERATIVE MANAGEMENT

- elevation, minimal weight bearing for 3–5 days
- crutches as needed with gradual progression in weight bearing and strengthening exercise

COMPLICATIONS

- infection
- wound dehiscence
- injury to any neurovascular structure in the leg
- recurrence of symptoms (uncommon)

SELECTED REFERENCES

Schepsis AA, Martini D, Corbett M. Surgical management of exertional compartment syndrome of the lower leg. Long-term followup. Am J Sports Med 1993; 21:811–817.
Blackman PG. A review of chronic exertional compartment syndrome in the lower leg. Med Sci Sports Exerc 2000;32:S4–10.

ARTHROTOMY, ANKLE, REMOVAL OF OSTEOPHYTES

CPT code   27640 arthrotomy, ankle (tibiotalar and fibulotalar
                    joints), surgical with removal of osteophytes

ICD-9 code   718.97 anterior ankle impingement

INDICATIONS

- chronic anterior ankle pain with dorsiflexion
- restricted dorsiflexion motion impairing push-off
- swelling
- failed conservative treatment
- lateral x-ray shows anterior osteophytes of tibial plafond and talar neck

ALTERNATIVE TREATMENTS

- nonoperative treatment
- arthroscopy, ankle

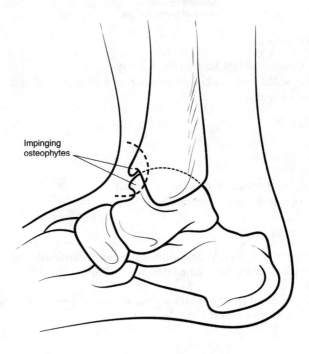

Impinging
osteophytes

APPROACHES

Surgical Techniques

- anteromedial incision: 2–3 cm in length just medial to tibialis anterior tendon
- protect saphenous vein, incise capsule longitudinally
- use ¼-inch, ½-inch osteotomes and rongeurs to resect osteophytes from talar neck, anterior tibia, and medial malleolus
- close capsule and skin in routine fashion
- anterolateral incision occasionally necessary to resect osteophytes from lateral tibia, talus, and fibula
- incision is longitudinal, lateral to extensor tendons and peroneus tertius
- protect lateral branch of superficial peroneal nerve
- incise capsule between medial border of fibula and lateral edge of talus
- use osteotomes and rongeurs to resect osteophytes and fibrous tissue

HIP, FOOT,
& ANKLE

POSTOPERATIVE MANAGEMENT

- elevation, non-weight-bearing for 3–5 days
- partial weight bearing, ROM exercises at 3–5 days (may vary depending on intra-articular procedure)
- accelerated ROM program to gain dorsiflexion

COMPLICATIONS

- infection
- synovial-cutaneous fistula
- sural, peroneal, saphenous nerve injury
- vascular injury

SELECTED REFERENCES

Scranton PE, Mc Dermott J. Anterior tibiotalar spurs: a comparison of open versus arthroscopic debridement. Foot Ankle 1992;13:125–129.
DiGiovanni BF, Fraga CJ, Cohen BE, Shereff MJ. Associated injuries found in chronic lateral ankle instability. Foot Ankle Int 2000;2:809–815.

NOTES

_____

_____

_____

_____

_____

REPAIR OF ACHILLES TENDON

CPT code   27650 repair of Achilles tendon

ICD-9 code   845.09 acute rupture of Achilles tendon

INDICATIONS

- high-demand patient (athlete, laborer)—return of strength important

ALTERNATIVE TREATMENTS

- nonoperative treatment, cast immobilization for minimum of 8 weeks
- percutaneous method

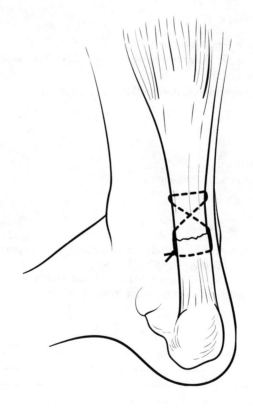

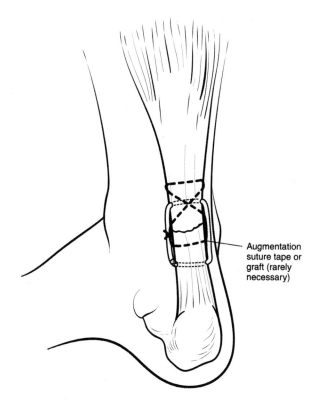

Augmentation suture tape or graft (rarely necessary)

APPROACHES

- prone position
- prepare both ankles so that the normal side can be used to compare and properly tension repair
- posterior incision just medial to midline
- do not create skin flaps

Surgical Techniques

- incise and reflect paratenon
- modified Kessler suture technique with no. 5 suture
- epitendon repair along repair margin with "0" absorbable suture

POSTOPERATIVE MANAGEMENT

- splint in equinus for 7–10 days
- short-leg cast for 4–6 weeks, progressively bringing foot to neutral, OR
- may begin early motion after first week limiting dorsiflexion past neutral using ankle-foot-orthosis or cast boot for 6 weeks
- begin strengthening at 6 weeks, no athletic activity for 4–6 months

COMPLICATIONS

- infection
- skin necrosis
- sural nerve injury
- re-rupture

SELECTED REFERENCES

Rebeccato A, Santini S, Salmaso G, Nogarin L. Repair of the Achilles tendon rupture: a comparison of three surgical techniques. J Foot Ankle Surg 2001;40:188–194.

Schepsis AA, Jones H, Haas AL. Achilles tendon disorders in athletes. Am J Sports Med 2002;30:287–305.

NOTES

_____

_____

_____

_____

_____

_____

_____

_____

_____

_____

_____

_____

_____

_____

HIP, FOOT,
& ANKLE

REPAIR OF ACHILLES TENDON, PERCUTANEOUS

CPT code   27650 percutaneous repair of Achilles tendon

ICD-9 code   845.09 acute rupture of Achilles tendon

INDICATIONS

- high-demand patient (athlete, laborer)—return of strength important
- open repair

ALTERNATIVE TREATMENTS

- nonoperative treatment with cast immobilization for minimum of 8 weeks

APPROACHES

- prone position
- prepare both ankles so that the normal side can be used to compare and properly tension repair

Surgical Techniques

- use Keith needle with no. 2 or 5 suture and puncture skin and traverse proximal portion of Achilles, 2–3 cm proximal to tear gap
- continue traversing in a criss-cross manner with each limb of suture to tear site
- use similar technique on distal segment starting 2–3 cm distal to gap
- tunnel medially and laterally to retrieve sutures on each side of tear and tie under appropriate tension

POSTOPERATIVE MANAGEMENT

- splint in equinus for 7–10 days
- short-leg cast for 4–6 weeks, progressively bringing foot to neutral, OR
- may begin early motion after first week limiting dorsiflexion past neutral using an ankle-foot orthosis or cast boot for 6 weeks
- begin strengthening at 6 weeks, no athletic activity for 4–6 months

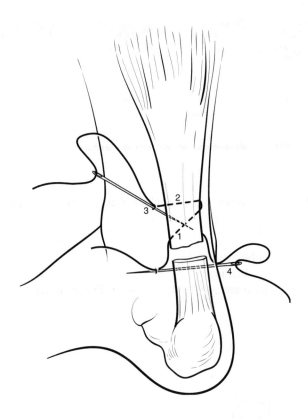

HIP, FOOT, & ANKLE

COMPLICATIONS

- infection
- skin necrosis
- sural nerve injury
- re-rupture

SELECTED REFERENCES

Ma GW, Griffith TG. Percutaneous repair of acute closed ruptures of the Achilles tendon: a new technique. Clin Orthop 1977;128:247–255.

Assal M, Jung M, Stern R, Rippstein P, Delmi M, Hoffmeyer P. Limited open repair of Achilles tendon ruptures: a technique with a new instrument and findings of a prospective multicenter study. J Bone Joint Surg Am 2002; 84-A:161–170.

REPAIR, DISLOCATING PERONEAL TENDONS WITHOUT FIBULAR OSTEOTOMY

CPT code   27675 repair, dislocating peroneal tendons without
                            fibular osteotomy

ICD-9 code   854.10 subluxation/dislocation, peroneal tendons

INDICATIONS

- subluxation or dislocation of peroneal tendons, acute or chronic/recurrent

ALTERNATIVE TREATMENTS

- acute—cast immobilization
- chronic/recurrent—bracing
- repair with fibular osteotomy or deepening of fibular groove

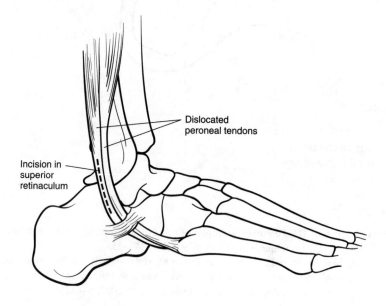

Dislocated
peroneal tendons

Incision in
superior
retinaculum

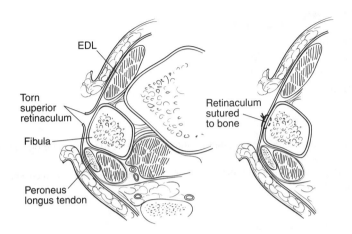

SURGICAL ANATOMY

Incision

- longitudinal incision over distal fibula
- incise retinaculum just posterior to fibula cortex

APPROACHES

- many procedures described
- procedure selection dependent on anatomy
- lateral or semilateral position
- incision over peroneal sheath posterior to distal fibula
- repairs—repair the superior peroneal retinaculum back to the fibula

Surgical Techniques

- techniques—suture to periosteum, suture through drill holes, suture using suture anchors in fibula (retinaculum frequently stripped with periosteum so that a Bankart-type repair can be done)
- reconstructions—reconstruct superior peroneal retinaculum with soft tissue, described procedures include use of: fibular periosteum, part of Achilles tendon, part of peroneus brevis tendon, calcaneofibular ligament, plantaris tendon

POSTOPERATIVE MANAGEMENT

- short-leg walking cast for 6–8 weeks
- weight bearing important to prevent adhesions

COMPLICATIONS

- infection
- recurrent subluxation
- peroneal tendon adhesions
- sural nerve injury

SELECTED REFERENCES

Brage ME, Hansen ST Jr. Traumatic subluxation/dislocation of the peroneal tendons. Foot Ankle 1992;13:423–431.

Mann RA. Subluxation and dislocation of the peroneal tendons. Op Tech Sports Med 1999;7:2–6.

NOTES

_____

_____

_____

_____

_____

_____

_____

_____

_____

_____

HIP, FOOT,
& ANKLE

REPAIR, DISLOCATING PERONEAL TENDONS WITH FIBULAR OSTEOTOMY

CPT code   27676 repair, dislocating peroneal tendons with
                       fibular osteotomy

ICD-9 code   854.10 subluxation/dislocation, peroneal tendons

INDICATIONS

- subluxation or dislocation of peroneal tendons, acute or chronic/recurrent

ALTERNATIVE TREATMENTS

- acute—cast immobilization
- chronic/recurrent—bracing
- soft tissue repair without osteotomy

APPROACHES

Surgical Techniques
- many procedures described
- procedure selection dependent on anatomy
- osteotomy or fibular deepening if soft tissues are inadequate or if convex/shallow fibular floor of peroneal tunnel
- lateral or semi-lateral position
- incision over peroneal sheath posterior to distal fibula
- bony procedures:
  - deepening of fibular groove
    - remove cancellous bone through cortical window and then compress cortex
    - reattach peroneal tendon sheath to fibula through periosteum sutures, drill holes, or suture anchor
  - fibular osteotomies
    - rotational osteotomies
    - sliding osteotomies
      - horizontal—DeVries
      - vertical—Micheli

POSTOPERATIVE MANAGEMENT

- short-leg walking cast for 6–8 weeks
- weight bearing important to prevent adhesions

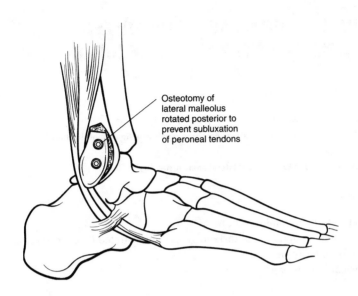

Osteotomy of
lateral malleolus
rotated posterior to
prevent subluxation
of peroneal tendons

HIP, FOOT,
& ANKLE

COMPLICATIONS

- infection
- recurrent subluxation
- fibula/osteotomy fracture
- peroneal tendon adhesions
- sural nerve injury

SELECTED REFERENCES

Brage ME, Hansen ST Jr. Traumatic subluxation/dislocation of the peroneal tendons. Foot Ankle 1992;13:423–431.
Jones DC. Tendon disorders of the foot and ankle. J Am Acad Orthop Surg 1993; 1:87–94.

NOTES

REPAIR, SECONDARY, DISRUPTED LIGAMENT, LATERAL ANKLE (BROSTROM REPAIR WITH GOULD MODIFICATION)

CPT code 27696 repair, secondary, disrupted ligament(s)
ankle, lateral, Brostrom repair with Gould modification

ICD-9 code 718.87 recurrent lateral ankle instability

INDICATIONS

- recurrent lateral ankle sprains
- mechanical lateral ankle instability as demonstrated by excessive talar tilt and/or anterior drawer
- normal hind foot alignment

ALTERNATIVE TREATMENTS

- rehabilitation emphasizing strengthening and proprioception
- ankle taping and/or bracing
- Brostrom repair with modified Evans tenodesis
- other lateral ankle reconstructions (Chrisman-Snook, Watson-Jones, Elmslie, etc.)

APPROACHES

- lateral or semi-lateral position
- curvilinear incision following the anterior and distal contour of the distal fibula or oblique incision over distal fibula and lateral foot

Surgical Techniques

- incise lateral ankle capsule, including anterior talofibular (ATF) ligament, adjacent to fibula
- incise peroneal sheath and retract tendons
- identify calcaneofibular (CF) ligament and incise adjacent to fibula
- excise redundancy in ATF and CF ligaments
- repair ligaments to periosteum with braided, nonabsorbable no. 2 suture
- advance extensor retinaculum superiorly, and suture over ligament repair to periosteum of distal fibula (Gould modification—designed to limit subtalar inversion)

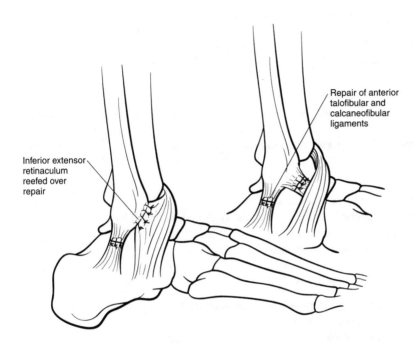

Repair of anterior talofibular and calcaneofibular ligaments

Inferior extensor retinaculum reefed over repair

HIP, FOOT, & ANKLE

POSTOPERATIVE MANAGEMENT

- splint for 10–14 days
- short-leg walking cast or CAM walker for 4 weeks
- air stirrup for 4 weeks
- start ROM and strengthening at 6 weeks
- return to full activity at 3–4 months

COMPLICATIONS

- infection
- hematoma
- injury to sural or superficial peroneal nerves and their branches
- recurrent instability

SELECTED REFERENCES

Gould N, Seligson D, Gassman J. Early and late repair of the lateral ligaments of the ankle. Foot Ankle 1980;1:84–89.

Hamilton WG, Thompson FM, Snow SW. The modified Brostrom procedure for lateral ankle instability. Foot Ankle 1993;14:1–7.

REPAIR, SECONDARY, DISRUPTED LIGAMENT, LATERAL ANKLE (BROSTROM REPAIR)

CPT code   27696 repair, secondary, disrupted ligament(s) ankle, lateral, Brostrom repair

ICD-9 code   718.87 recurrent lateral ankle instability

INDICATIONS

- recurrent lateral ankle sprains
- mechanical lateral ankle instability as demonstrated by excessive talar tilt and/or anterior drawer
- normal hind foot alignment

ALTERNATIVE TREATMENTS

- rehabilitation emphasizing strengthening and proprioception
- ankle taping and/or bracing
- Brostrom repair with modified Evans tenodesis
- other lateral ankle reconstructions (Chrisman-Snook, Watson-Jones, Elmslie, etc.)

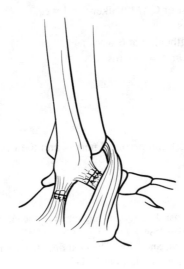

APPROACHES

- lateral or semi-lateral position
- curvilinear incision following the anterior and distal contour of the distal fibula or oblique incision over distal fibula and lateral foot

Surgical Techniques

- incise lateral ankle capsule, including anterior talofibular (ATF) ligament, adjacent to fibula
- incise peroneal sheath and retract tendons
- identify calcaneofibular (CF) ligament and incise adjacent to fibula
- excise redundancy in ATF and CF ligaments
- repair ligaments to periosteum with braided, nonabsorbable no. 2 suture
- advance extensor retinaculum superiorly and suture over ligament repair to periosteum of distal fibula (Gould modification—designed to limit subtalar inversion)

HIP, FOOT, & ANKLE

POSTOPERATIVE MANAGEMENT

- splint for 10–14 days
- short-leg walking cast or CAM walker for 4 weeks
- air stirrup for 4 weeks
- start ROM and strengthening at 6 weeks
- return to full activity at 3–4 months

COMPLICATIONS

- infection
- hematoma
- injury to sural or superficial peroneal nerves and their branches
- recurrent instability

SELECTED REFERENCES

Gould N, Seligson D, Gassman J. Early and late repair of the lateral ligaments of the ankle. Foot Ankle 1980;1:84–89.
Hamilton WG, Thompson FM, Snow SW. The modified Brostrom procedure for lateral ankle instability. Foot Ankle 1993;14:1–7.

NOTES

_____
_____
_____
_____
_____

REPAIR, SECONDARY, DISRUPTED LIGAMENT, LATERAL ANKLE (BROSTROM WITH MODIFIED EVANS TENODESIS)

CPT code   27698 repair, secondary, disrupted ligament(s) ankle, lateral, Brostrom repair
with modified Evans tenodesis

ICD-9 codes   718.87 recurrent lateral ankle instability

INDICATIONS

- same as Brostrom repair with Gould modification
- additional restraint to excessive subtalar inversion

ALTERNATIVE TREATMENTS

- rehabilitation emphasizing strengthening and proprioception
- ankle taping and/or bracing
- Brostrom repair with Gould modification
- other lateral ankle reconstructions (Chrisman-Snook, Watson-Jones, Elmslie, etc.)

APPROACHES

- same steps as Brostrom repair with Gould modification, plus tenodesis with one half of peroneus brevis
- oblique incision over distal fibula and lateral foot

Surgical Techniques

- longitudinally split the peroneus brevis in half, and:
- preserve superior peroneal retinaculum
- proximally transect tendon-half with the least attachment to muscle belly
- pull out tendon distally leaving insertion intact
- place passing suture in end of tendon
- pass tendon graft through 4–6 mm drill hole between ATF and CF insertions, exiting 2–3 cm proximally at posterior fibula
- fix graft halfway between full eversion and full inversion to act as a check rein against inversion and to protect ligament repair
- suture graft to fibular periosteum with no. 2 nonabsorbable suture

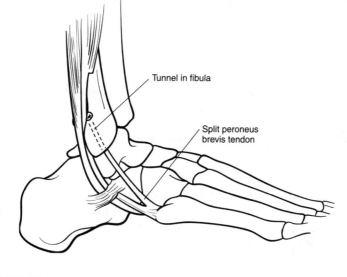

Tunnel in fibula

Split peroneus brevis tendon

POSTOPERATIVE MANAGEMENT

- same as Brostrom repair with Gould modification
- start ROM and strengthening at 6 weeks
- return to full activity at 3–4 months

COMPLICATIONS

- infection
- hematoma
- injury to sural or superficial peroneal nerves and their branches
- recurrent instability

SELECTED REFERENCE

Girard P, Anderson RB, Davis WH, Isear JA, Kiebzak GM. Clinical evaluation of the modified Brostrom-Evans procedure to restore ankle instability. Foot Ankle 1999;4:246–252.

NOTES

_____

_____

_____

_____

_____

_____

REPAIR, SECONDARY, DISRUPTED LIGAMENT, LATERAL ANKLE (CHRISMAN-SNOOK PROCEDURE)

CPT code   27698 repair, secondary, disrupted ligament(s), ankle, lateral, Chrisman-Snook procedure

ICD-9 code   718.87 recurrent lateral ankle instability

INDICATIONS

- same as Brostrom repair with Gould modification
- absence of repairable anterior talofibular and/or calcaneofibular ligaments
- should be used sparingly as this procedure is nonanatomic and can significantly restrict subtalar motion

ALTERNATIVE TREATMENTS

- nonoperative treatments—see Brostrom repairs
- Brostrom repair with Gould modification
- Brostrom repair with modified Evans tenodesis
- other lateral ankle reconstructions (Watson-Jones, Elmslie, Evans, etc.)

APPROACHES

- lateral or semi-lateral position
- oblique incision over distal fibula and lateral foot or long curved incision over peroneal tendons

Surgical Techniques

- repair any remaining ligament tissue
- harvest one half of peroneus brevis tendon (see Brostrom repair with modified Evans tenodesis)
- drill anterior to posterior hole, approximately 6 mm in diameter, just proximal to ankle joint
- pass graft through fibula and suture to periosteum with foot and ankle in neutral position
- make lateral calcaneal bone tunnel by connecting two drill holes
- pass graft over remaining peroneus brevis and peroneus longus tendons
- pass graft from posterior to anterior through calcaneal tunnel with foot and ankle in neutral position.
- suture remaining graft to anterior limb of repair

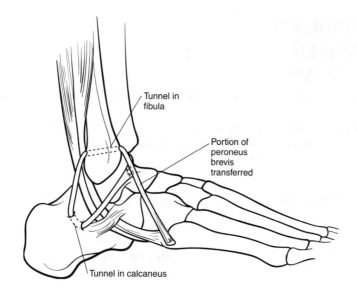

POSTOPERATIVE MANAGEMENT

- same as Brostrom repair with Gould modification

COMPLICATIONS

- infection
- hematoma
- injury to sural or superficial peroneal nerves and their branches
- recurrent instability
- subtalar stiffness, loss of motion

SELECTED REFERENCES

Chrisman OD, Snook GA. Reconstruction of lateral ligament tears of the ankle. J Bone Joint Surg 1969;51A:904–912.

Snook GA, Wilson TC. Long-term results of the Chrisman-Snook operation for reconstruction of the lateral ligaments of the ankle. J Bone Joint Surg 1985; 67A:1–7.

NOTES

INTERNAL FIXATION OF DISTAL TIBIOFIBULAR JOINT

CPT code   27829 internal fixation of distal tibiofibular joint (syndesmosis) disruption

ICD-9 codes   824.2 Maisonneuve fracture

     837, 845.0 Grade III syndesmosis sprain

INDICATIONS

- unstable syndesmosis after ligamentous injury with or without fracture

ALTERNATIVE TREATMENTS

- closed, nonoperative treatment (long-leg cast immobilization)

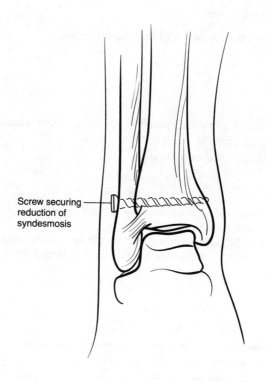

Screw securing reduction of syndesmosis

APPROACHES

Surgical Techniques

- closed reduction by placement of large clamp on medial and lateral malleoli through skin
- if associated distal fibula fracture, screw can be placed through distal screw-hole of plate
- ankle in maximal dorsiflexion
- drill and tap four cortices parallel and approximately 1 cm proximal to ankle joint, and orient drill obliquely from posterolateral to anteromedial in line with intermalleolar axis
- fixation with 4.5-mm cortical screw across four cortices

POSTOPERATIVE MANAGEMENT

- splint for 10–14 days
- partial weight bearing in cast boot or short-leg cast for 4–6 weeks—may advance to full weight bearing in some cases
- screw removal after 3 months

COMPLICATIONS

- infection
- loss of ankle motion
- screw breakage
- fracture after screw removal
- tibiofibular synostosis

SELECTED REFERENCES

Clanton TO, Paul P: Syndesmosis injuries in athletes. Foot Ankle Clin 2002 September;7(3):529–549.

Wuest TK. Injuries to the distal lower extremity syndesmosis. J Am Acad Orthop Surg 1997;5:172,181.

NOTES

_____

_____

_____

_____

_____

_____

_____

_____

HIP, FOOT,
& ANKLE

INTERNAL FIXATION, FIFTH METATARSAL FRACTURE

CPT code   27829 internal fixation fifth metatarsal fracture

ICD-9 code   825.25 fifth metatarsal fracture

INDICATION

- metadiaphyseal fracture of fifth metatarsal

ALTERNATIVE TREATMENTS

- closed, nonoperative treatment, non-weight-bearing for 6 weeks

APPROACHES

- supine or lateral decubitus
- use mini-flouro or C-arm image
- 1–2 cm incision extending proximally from base of the fifth styloid

Surgical Techniques

- use 3.2 mm drill starting at base and aiming for center of fifth metatarsal intrameduallary canal
- verify center position on anteroposterior and lateral images
- tap proximal fragment with 4.5 mm tap
- use 4.5 mm malleolar or 6.5 AO cancellous screw
- place screw and verify position by x-ray

POSTOPERATIVE MANAGEMENT

- splint for 10–14 days
- partial weight bearing in cast boot or short-leg cast for 4–6 weeks—may advance to full weight bearing in some cases

COMPLICATIONS

- infection
- non-union
- hardware pain

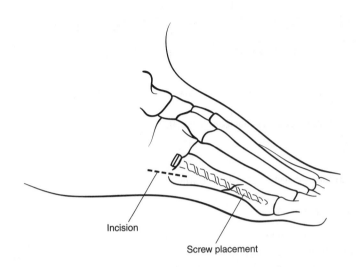

Incision

Screw placement

HIP, FOOT,
& ANKLE

SELECTED REFERENCES

DeLee JC, Evans JP, Julian J. Stress fracture of the fifth metatarsal. Am J Sports Med 1983;11:349–353.

Rosenberg GA, Sferra JJ. Treatment strategies for acute fractures and nonunions of the proximal fifth metatarsal. J Am Acad Orthop Surg 2000;8:332–338.

NOTES

ARTHROSCOPY, ANKLE—DEBRIDEMENT, CURETTAGE, OR DRILLING OF TALUS

CPT code   29891 ankle arthroscopy, debridement, curettage or drilling of talus

ICD-9 code   732.7 osteochondral lesion of the talus

INDICATIONS

- osteochondral lesions of the talar dome

ALTERNATIVE TREATMENTS

- nonoperative treatment
- autograft or allograft transfer for large lesions
- ankle arthrodesis (large lesions with marked osteoarthrosis)

APPROACHES

Surgical Techniques
- lateral lesions—ankle arthroscopy
  - debride localized synovitis
  - remove ostoechondal lesion
  - curettage, drilling, or microfracture base of lesion

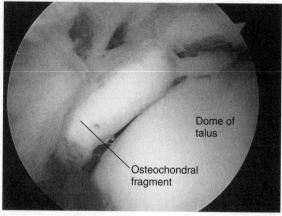

Dome of talus

Osteochondral fragment

Right ankle—displaced lateral dome osteochondrial fracture

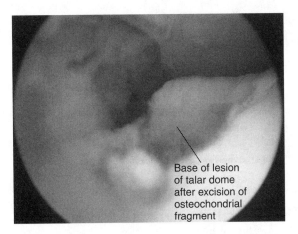

Base of lesion of talar dome after excision of osteochondrial fragment

- medial lesion—usually requires approach through medial malleolar osteotomy
  - predrill for one or two malleolar screws
  - oblique osteotomy at medial corner of mortise with thin osteotome or saw blade
  - protect tibialis posterior tendon
  - fix with one or two malleolar screws at conclusion of procedure
  - curettage, drilling, or microfracture base of lesion
  - second option: transmalleolar drilling through medial malleolus to approach posteromedial lesion

POSTOPERATIVE MANAGEMENT

- dependent on graft type

COMPLICATIONS

- infection
- continued pain, arthrosis
- incongruous articular surface
- medial malleolar non-union/malunion
- neurovascular injury

SELECTED REFERENCES

Stone JW. Osteochondral lesions of the talar dome. J Am Acad Orthop Surg 1996; 4:63–73.

Ogilvie-Harris DJ, Sarrosa EA. Arthroscopic treatment of osteochondritis dissecans of the talus. Arthroscopy 1999;8:805–808.

Kumai T, Takakura Y, Higashiyama I, Tamai S. Arthroscopic drilling for the treatment of osteochondral lesions of the talus. J Bone Joint Surg Am 1999;81:1229–1235.

ARTHROSCOPY, ANKLE (TIBIOTALAR AND FIBULOTALAR), SURGICAL, WITH DEBRIDEMENT

CPT code   **29897 arthroscopy, ankle (tibiotalar and fibulotalar joints), surgical, with debridement**

ICD-9 code   **718.97 chronic ankle impingement**

INDICATIONS

- chronic anterior-lateral ankle pain after inversion injury
- tenderness over lateral ligaments
- no instability
- failed conservative treatment including ankle rehabilitation

ALTERNATIVE TREATMENTS

- nonoperative treatment
- arthrotomy, ankle

SURGICAL ANATOMY

Incision

Soft tissue
impingement
lesion

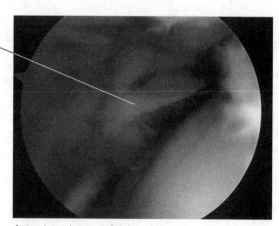

Anterolateral gutter of right ankle

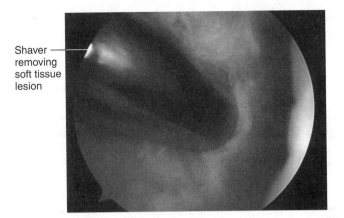

Shaver removing soft tissue lesion

APPROACHES

Surgical Techniques

- may use standard 4.0-mm 30° or 2.7-mm 30° arthroscope—depending on preference, joint space size
- ankle joint distension with saline/Ringer's lactate
- gravity or noninvasive distraction device
- incise only skin to make portals, blunt dissection with clamp to capsule
  - for anteromedial portal—tibialis anterior—saphenous vein interval, introduce arthroscope in this portal
  - for anterolateral portal—lateral to peroneus tertius, EDL tendons, avoid branches of superficial peroneal nerve

POSTOPERATIVE MANAGEMENT

- elevation, non-weight-bearing for 3–5 days
- partial weight bearing, ROM exercises at 3–5 days (may vary depending on intra-articular procedure).

COMPLICATIONS

- infection
- synovial-cutaneous fistula
- sural, peroneal, saphenous nerve injury
- vascular injury

SELECTED REFERENCES

Stetson WB, Ferkel RD. Ankle arthroscopy: I. Technique and complications. J Am Acad Orthop Surg 1996;4:17–23.
Stetson WB, Ferkel RD. Ankle arthroscopy: II. Indications and results. J Am Acad Orthop Surg 1996;4:24–33.

ARTHROSCOPY, ANKLE, WITH REMOVAL OF OSTEOPHYTES

CPT code   **29898** arthroscopy, ankle (tibiotalar and fibulotalar joints), surgical with removal of osteophytes

ICD-9 code   **718.97** anterior ankle impingement

INDICATIONS

- chronic anterior ankle pain with dorsiflexion
- restricted dorsiflexion motion impairing push-off
- swelling
- failed conservative treatment
- lateral x-ray shows anterior osteophytes of tibial plafond and talar neck

ALTERNATIVE TREATMENTS

- nonoperative treatment
- arthrotomy, ankle

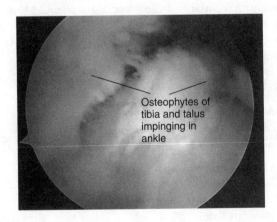

Osteophytes of tibia and talus impinging in ankle

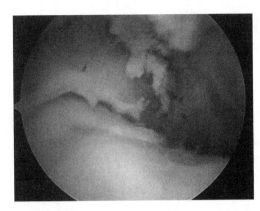

Osteophytes
removed

SURGICAL APPROACHES

Surgical Techniques

- may use standard 4.0-mm 30° or 2.7-mm 30° arthroscope, depending on preference and joint space size
- ankle joint distension with saline/Ringer's lactate
- gravity or noninvasive distraction device
- incise only skin to make portals, blunt dissection with clamp to capsule
  - anteromedial portal—tibialis anterior-saphenous vein interval (introduce arthroscope in this portal)
  - anterolateral portal—lateral to peroneus tertius, EDL tendons (avoid branches of superficial peroneal nerve)
  - use shaver, burr, or osteotome to remove anterior osteophytes
  - verify resection with C-arm or mini-scan

POSTOPERATIVE MANAGEMENT

- elevation, non-weight-bearing for 3–5 days
- partial weight bearing, ROM exercises at 3–5 days (may vary depending on intra-articular procedure).

COMPLICATIONS

- infection
- synovial-cutaneous fistula
- sural, peroneal, saphenous nerve injury
- vascular injury

SELECTED REFERENCES

Stetson WB, Ferkel RD. Ankle arthroscopy: I. Technique and complications. J Am Acad Orthop Surg 1996;4:17–23.

Tol JL, Verheyen CP, van Dijk CN. Arthroscopic treatment of anterior impingement of the ankle. J Bone Joint Surg Br 2001;83:9–13.

ARTHROSCOPY, ANKLE (TIBIOTALAR AND FIBULOTALAR), SURGICAL

CPT code 29891, 29894, 29895, 29897, 29898 arthroscopy, ankle (tibiotalar and
fibulotalar joints), surgical

ICD-9 code(s) **718.17** loose body
        718.37 internal derangement
        732.7 osteochondritis dessecans

INDICATIONS

- arthritis infectious disease (711.87)
- symptomatic loose body or foreign body (718.17)
- painful ankle after ankle sprain with soft tissue impingement (718.97)
- chronic pain, swelling of ankle (719.47)
- painful or displaced talar dome fracture (845.21)

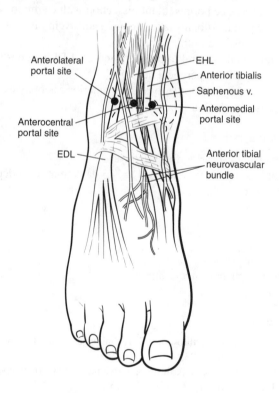

Anterolateral portal site   EHL

Anterior tibialis

Saphenous v.

Anterocentral portal site   Anteromedial portal site

EDL

Anterior tibial neurovascular bundle

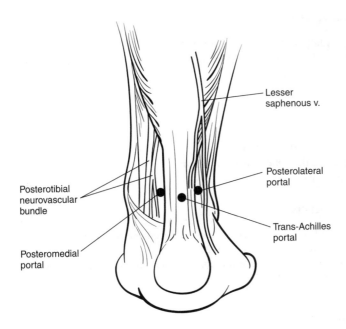

Lesser saphenous v.

Posterolateral portal

Posterotibial neurovascular bundle

Trans-Achilles portal

Posteromedial portal

ALTERNATIVE TREATMENTS

- nonoperative treatment
- arthrotomy, ankle

APPROACHES

Surgical Techniques

- may use standard 4.0-mm 30° or 2.7-mm 30° arthroscope, depending on preference and joint space size
- ankle joint distension with saline/Ringer's lactate
- gravity or noninvasive distraction device
- incise only skin to make portals, blunt dissection with clamp to capsule
- anteromedial portal—tibialis anterior-saphenous vein interval (introduce arthroscope in this portal)
- anterolateral portal—lateral to peroneus tertius, EDL tendons (avoid branches of superficial peroneal nerve)
- posterolateral portal—just lateral to Achilles tendon
- use shaver to debride fibrous tissue or synovitis
- remove transchondral lesion and drill or curette base to promote bleeding and fibrocartilage repair

POSTOPERATIVE MANAGEMENT

- elevation, non-weight-bearing for 3–5 days
- partial weight bearing, ROM exercises at 3–5 days (may vary depending on intra-articular procedure).

COMPLICATIONS

- infection
- synovial-cutaneous fistula
- sural, peroneal, saphenous nerve injury
- vascular injury

SELECTED REFERENCES

Stetson WB, Ferkel RD. Ankle arthroscopy: I. Technique and complications. J Am Acad Orthop Surg 1996;4:17–23.

Stetson WB, Ferkel RD. Ankle arthroscopy: II. Indications and results. J Am Acad Orthop Surg 1996;4:24–33.

NOTES

_____

_____

_____

_____

_____

_____

_____

_____

_____

_____

_____

_____

BONE GRAFTING, OSTEOCHONDRAL LESION OF THE TALUS

CPT code   **29999** **open autograft bone grafting, osteochondral lesion of the talus**
open allograft bone grafting, osteochondral lesion of the talus
autograft osteochondral grafting, osteochondral lesion of the talus
(OATS or mosaicplasty procedures)
allograft osteochondral grafting, osteochondral lesion of the talus
autologous chondrocyte transplantation, osteochondral lesion
of the talus

ICD-9 code   **732.7** **osteochondral lesion of the talus**

INDICATIONS

- large osteochondral lesions of the talar dome
- pain, swelling, disability not responsive to conservative treatment

ALTERNATIVE TREATMENTS

- nonoperative treatment
- ankle arthrodesis (large lesions with marked osteoarthrosis)

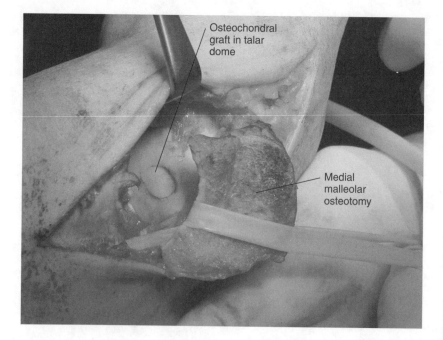

Osteochondral graft in talar dome

Medial malleolar osteotomy

APPROACHES

Surgical Techniques

- lateral lesions—anterolateral arthrotomy: may require removal of localized area of anterior-lateral tibial plafond
- medial lesion—usually requires approach through medial malleolar osteotomy
  - pre-drill for one or two malleolar screws
  - oblique osteotomy at medial corner of mortise with thin osteotome or saw blade
  - protect tibialis posterior tendon
  - fix with one or two malleolar screws at conclusion of procedure
- curretage of lesion
- implant of graft—dependent on procedure

HIP, FOOT, & ANKLE

POSTOPERATIVE MANAGEMENT

- dependent on graft type

COMPLICATIONS

- infection
- loosening of graft
- incongruous articular surface
- medial malleolar non-union/malunion
- neurovascular injury

SELECTED REFERENCES

Stone JW. Osteochondral lesions of the talar dome. J Am Acad Orthop Surg 1996;4:63–73.

Hangody L, Kish G, Modis L, Szerb I, Gaspar L, Dioszegi Z, Kendik Z. Mosaic-plasty for the treatment of osteochondritis dissecans of the talus: two to seven year results in 36 patients. Foot Ankle Int 2001;22:552–558.

Giannini S, Buda R, Grigolo B, Vannini F. Autologous chondrocyte transplantation in osteochondral lesions of the ankle joint. Foot Ankle Int 2001;22:513–517.

Gross AE, Agnidis Z, Hutchison CR. Osteochondral defects of the talus treated with fresh osteochondral allograft transplantation. Foot Ankle Int 2001;22:385–391.

NOTES

_____

_____

_____

_____

_____

INDEX

Page references followed by f indicate figures.